DEJA REVIEW™

Neuroscience

NOTICE

Medicine is an ever-changing science. As new research and clinical experience broaden our knowledge, changes in treatment and drug therapy are required. The authors and the publisher of this work have checked with sources believed to be reliable in their efforts to provide information that is complete and generally in accord with the standards accepted at the time of publication. However, in view of the possibility of human error or changes in medical sciences, neither the authors nor the publisher nor any other party who has been involved in the preparation or publication of this work warrants that the information contained herein is in every respect accurate or complete, and they disclaim all responsibility for any errors or omissions or for the results obtained from use of the information contained in this work. Readers are encouraged to confirm the information contained herein with other sources. For example and in particular, readers are advised to check the product information sheet included in the package of each drug they plan to administer to be certain that the information contained in this work is accurate and that changes have not been made in the recommended dose or in the contraindications for administration. This recommendation is of particular importance in connection with new or infrequently used drugs.

DEJA REVIEW™

Neuroscience

Second Edition

Matthew Tremblay

MD/PhD Candidate
Medical Scientist Training Program
Albert Einstein College of Medicine
Bronx, New York

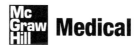 Medical

New York   Chicago   San Francisco   Lisbon   London   Madrid   Mexico City
Milan   New Delhi   San Juan   Seoul   Singapore   Sydney   Toronto

Deja Review™: Neuroscience, Second Edition

1 2 3 4 5 6 7 8 9   DOC/DOC   14 13 12 11 10

ISBN 978-0-07-162727-6
MHID 0-07-162727-8

This book was set in Palatino by Glyph International.
The editor was Kirsten Funk.
The production supervisor was Catherine Saggese.
Project management was provided by Preeti Longia Sinha of Glyph International.
RR Donnelly was the printer and binder.

This book is printed on acid-free paper.

Library of Congress Cataloging-in-Publication Data

Tremblay, Matthew.
    Deja review : neuroscience / Matthew Tremblay.—2nd ed.
       p. ; cm.—(Deja review)
    Includes index.
    ISBN 978-0-07-162727-6 (pbk. : alk. paper)   1. Neurosciences—Examinations, questions, etc.   2. Nervous system—Diseases—Examinations, questions, etc.
I. Title.   II. Title: Neuroscience.   III. Series: Deja review.
    [DNLM: 1. Nervous System—Examination Questions.   2. Nervous System Diseases—Examination Questions.   WL 18.2 T789d   2010]
    RC343.6.T74   2010
    616.80076—dc22
                              2009034031

*To my parents, who taught me to pursue my dreams;
to family and friends, for their support and encouragement;
and to all of my teachers, for sharing the gift of knowledge.*

Contents

Faculty Advisor

Conwell H. Anderson, PhD
Associate Professor
Department of Anatomy and Cell Biology
University of Illinois at Chicago
Chicago, Illinois

Student Reviewers

Benjamin Han
SUNY Upstate Medical University
Class of 2009

Joshua Lynch
Lake Erie College of Osteopathic Medicine
Class of 2008

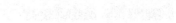

Contributing Author

David Snetman
Medical Student
Albert Einstein College of Medicine
Bronx, New York
Neuropharmacology

Contributing Authors to First Edition

Piyush Banker, MD
Albert Einstein College of Medicine
Class of 2007

Andrea Cotter, MD
Albert Einstein College of Medicine
Class of 2007

Jiwon Kim, MD
Albert Einstein College of Medicine
Class of 2007

Mark C. Liszewski, MD
Albert Einstein College of Medicine
Class of 2007

Will O'Brien, MD
Albert Einstein College of Medicine
Class of 2007

Rachel Ross
MD/PhD Candidate
Albert Einstein College of Medicine
Class of 2010

Joseph Stoklosa, MD
University of Pittsburgh
Class of 2007

Craig B. Woda, MD, PhD
Albert Einstein College of Medicine
Class of 2007

Preface

The *Deja Review* series is a unique resource that has been designed to allow you to review the essential facts and determine your level of knowledge on the subjects tested on Step 1 of the United States Medical Licensing Examination (USMLE). One of the major challenges of learning clinical neuroscience is integrating diverse knowledge ranging from the intricacies of neuroanatomy to the molecular cell biology of individual neurons. The Step 1 examination tests your understanding of basic science and pathology at all levels. Having taken Step 1, we felt it important to integrate anatomy, genetics, molecular biology, pathology, and pharmacology whenever possible.

ORGANIZATION

All concepts are presented in a question and answer format that covers key facts on commonly tested topics in medical neurosciences. The first chapters of the book are designed to review the fundamentals of basic neuroscience. From here, the focus shifts toward understanding neuroscience from a system's perspective. The final portion of the text explores pathologic states of the nervous system, with a particular emphasis on the molecular basis of disease. Chapters are organized into major classes of nervous system pathology. The compact, condensed design of the book is conducive to studying on the go, especially during any downtime throughout your day.

This question and answer format has several important advantages:

- It provides a rapid, straightforward way for you to assess your strengths and weaknesses.
- It allows you to efficiently review and commit to memory a large body of information.
- The vignettes found at the end of each chapter allow you to apply the facts you have just reviewed in a clinical scenario.
- It serves as a quick, last-minute review of high-yield facts.

In addition, a number of tables were included for rapid review of fundamental clinical and anatomic concepts. Anatomic drawings were included to illustrate basic neuroanatomy, a common Step 1 topic. Magnetic resonance (MRI) and computerized tomographic (CT) images were also incorporated to reflect a recent emphasis on imaging in the Step 1 examination.

HOW TO USE THIS BOOK

Remember, this text is not intended to replace comprehensive textbooks, course packs, or lectures. It is simply intended to serve as a supplement to your studies during your medical neuroscience course and Step 1 preparation. This text was contributed to by a number of medical students to represent the core topics tested on course examinations and Step 1. You may use the book to quiz yourself or classmates on topics covered in recent lectures and clinical case discussions.

However you choose to study, I hope you find this resource helpful throughout your preparation for course examinations and the USMLE Step 1.

Matthew Tremblay

Acknowledgments

First, I would like to thank the contributing authors of the current and previous editions of this text for taking time during clinical clerkships and laboratory research to help make this book a valuable resource. I would also like to thank the student and faculty reviewers for their thoughtful comments and helpful critiques. Special thanks to Dr. Michael L. Lipton, MD for providing a collection of important radiology images, as well as contributing his time and knowledge of anatomy and neuroradiology. I would also like to acknowledge the efforts of Judith R. Levin, Esq. for translating the enigmatic language of legalese. I need to thank Marsha Loeb, my previous acquisitions editor at McGraw-Hill, for recruiting me and helping me navigate the publishing process. My current acquisitions editor at McGraw-Hill, Kirsten Funk, deserves credit for helpful guidance in the process of completing this edition of the book and her persistence against procrastination. Finally, I need to thank my research advisor, Peter Davies, PhD, for his patience and understanding in allowing me to take time away from laboratory research and thesis writing to indulge my interest in teaching.

CHAPTER 1

Embryology and Histology

EMBRYOLOGY

Which region of the developing embryo becomes the neural plate?	Dorsal lip region
Invagination of the neural plate results in formation of what structure?	Neural groove
Neural folds on either side of the neural groove fuse to form what critical structure?	Neural tube
Neurulation takes place during what week of embryonic development?	Fourth week
An increase in what protein marker is often seen with neural tube defects?	α-Fetoprotein (AFP)
What disease is associated with low-maternal AFP?	Down syndrome
Caudal neural tube defects can be prevented by maternal consumption of what vitamin?	Folate
Which antiepileptic drug is associated with neural tube defects?	Valproic acid
Which groove separates the alar and basal plates?	Sulcus limitans
Which plate contains neurons with afferent functions (sensory)?	Dorsally located alar plate
Which plate contains neurons with efferent functions (motor)?	Ventrally located basal plate

| What are the three primary vesicles from rostral to caudal? | 1. Prosencephalon
2. Mesencephalon
3. Rhombencephalon |

Table 1.1 Embryologic Origins of CNS Structures

Primary Vesicle	Secondary Vesicle	Ventricle	Structure(s)
Prosencephalon	Telencephalon	Lateral ventricle	Cerebral hemispheres Limbic system Basal ganglia Corpus callosum Anterior commissure Olfactory nerve (CN I)
	Diencephalon	Third ventricle	Thalamus Hypothalamus Epithalamus Subthalamus Pineal body Optic nerve (CN II)

Mesencephalon	Mesencephalon	Cerebral aqueduct	Superior colliculus
			Inferior colliculus
			Cerebral peduncles
			Substantia nigra
			Nuclei of cranial nerves
			    Oculomotor (CN III)
			    Trochlear (CN IV)

Rhombencephalon	Metencephalon	Rostral fourth ventricle	Pons
			Cerebellum
			Nuclei of cranial nerves
			    Trigeminal (CN V)*
			    Abducens (CN VI)
			    Facial (CN VII)
			    Vestibulocochlear
			    (CN VIII)

	Myelencephalon	Caudal fourth ventricle	Medulla oblongata
			Nuclei of cranial nerves
			    Glossopharyngeal
			    (CN IX)
			    Vagus (CN X)
			    Hypoglossal (CN XII)

*Trigeminal nuclei can be found in the midbrain, pons, and medulla. The principal sensory and motor nuclei are located in the pons.

DIVISIONS OF THE NERVOUS SYSTEM

Which structures are considered part of the central nervous system (CNS)?	Brain, spinal cord, olfactory bulb and tract, optic nerve, and retina
What word describes collections of neuronal cell bodies in the CNS?	Nuclei
From which embryologic tissue are the cells of the CNS derived?	Neuroectoderm
Which structures make up the peripheral nervous system (PNS)?	Cranial nerves III-XII, spinal nerves, and autonomic ganglia and nerves
What word describes collections of neuronal cell bodies in the PNS?	Ganglia (*Exception:* Basal ganglia is a group of CNS nuclei.)
From which embryologic origin are the cells of the PNS derived?	Neural crest cells
What cell types and tissues are derived from neural crest cells?	Pseudounipolar neurons of peripheral ganglia, Schwann cells, neurons of autonomic ganglia, leptomeninges, chromaffin cells of adrenal medulla, melanocytes, odontoblasts, parafollicular C cells, pharyngeal arches, and aorticopulmonary septum
What are the three divisions of the autonomic nervous system (ANS)?	1. Sympathetic 2. Parasympathetic 3. Enteric
Which tissues are innervated by the ANS?	Smooth muscle, cardiac muscle, and glands
Which division of the ANS is responsible for the fight-or-flight response?	Sympathetic

NEUROHISTOLOGY

Which projections from neurons form complex arbors and receive afferent input?	Dendrites
What are the regions of the dendrite containing a high density of receptors?	Dendritic spines

What common cause of mental retardation is associated with malformation of dendritic spines?	Fragile X syndrome
What is the name of the projections from neurons that end in synaptic terminals?	Axons
What is the name of the region of the axon in which action potentials are generated?	Initial segment or axon hillock
What is another name for a neuronal cell body?	Soma
Nissl substance describes which neuronal organelles?	Ribosomes and rough endoplasmic reticulum
Which type of axonal transport uses dynein motors?	Fast retrograde transport
Which type of axonal transport uses kinesin motors?	Fast anterograde transport
Along which cytoskeletal elements do dynein and kinesin motors travel?	Microtubules

Name the type of neuron described below:

Neuron with unidirectional axon found in the peripheral ganglia	Pseudounipolar
Neuron with a single dendrite and an axon, common to the retina	Bipolar
Neuron with triangular shape and large apical dendrites found primarily in the cortex	Pyramidal
Cerebellar neuron with extensive planar dendritic arborization	Purkinje
Which cells are the major support cells of the CNS?	Astrocytes
What are the major functions of astrocytes?	Maintain ionic gradient Reuptake certain neurotransmitters Detoxify ammonia Secrete neurotrophic factors
Which protein is used as a cell-specific marker for astrocytes?	Glial fibrillary acidic protein (GFAP)

What word is used to describe the astrocytic response to injury, which leaves a scar in the brain?	Gliosis
What is the name used to describe the accumulations of heat shock proteins and filaments seen in reactive astrocytes?	Rosenthal fibers
What is the name of the fatty wrapping around axons which increases conduction velocity?	Myelin
What is the name for the gaps between myelin wrapping in which one finds a high density of sodium channels?	Nodes of Ranvier
Which cell type produces myelin in the CNS?	Oligodendroglia
Infection of oligodendroglia by the JC virus results in what disease?	Progressive multifocal leukoencephalopathy (see Chap. 12)
Which cell type produces myelin in the PNS?	Schwann cells
Do Schwann cells wrap unmyelinated peripheral axons?	Yes
Which cell type is capable of wrapping multiple axons?	Oligodendroglia
Which cell type wraps only single axons?	Schwann cells
Which CNS cells of mesodermal origin express the MHC II (major histocompatibility complex II) molecule, and act as the resident macrophages of the CNS?	Microglia
Microglia are heavily implicated in CNS pathology associated with infection by what virus?	HIV
What is the major function of microglia following CNS injury?	Phagocytosis of debris, including dead or dying neurons
Which type of cells line the ventricles?	Ependymal cells
Cerebrospinal fluid (CSF) is produced in what structure?	Choroid plexus

BLOOD-BRAIN BARRIER

What are the major components of the blood-brain barrier?	Nonfenestrated capillaries Endothelial tight junctions Astrocytic endfeet
What is the major determinant of whether a drug will readily cross the blood-brain barrier?	Lipid solubility
What kind of molecules are capable of crossing the blood-brain barrier?	Water Gases Lipid-soluble molecules Glucose (facilitative diffusion via Glut1 transporter) Amino acids (both passive and active transporters)
What is the generic term for midline structures of the brain lacking the blood-brain barrier?	Circumventricular organs
Name the circumventricular organs.	Pineal gland, median eminence, area postrema, subfornical organ, and subcommissural organ
Which circumventricular organ is responsible for vomiting in response to toxin consumption?	Area postrema, bordering the fourth ventricle

CORTICAL ORGANIZATION

What are the six layers of the cortex from outside to inside?	I: molecular layer II: external granular layer III: external pyramidal layer IV: internal granular layer V: internal pyramidal layer VI: multiform layer
Name the cortical layer described below:	
Primarily a receptive layer, made up of stellate neurons, predominant in sensory areas	Layer IV

Projects mostly to subcortical areas or spinal cord, made up of pyramidal neurons, predominant in motor areas	Layer V
Projects to other cortical areas	Layer III
Projects to the thalamus to maintain corticothalamic feedback	Layer VI

CHAPTER 2

Spinal Cord

Identify the labeled structures in the diagram of the cervical spinal cord (Fig. 2.1).

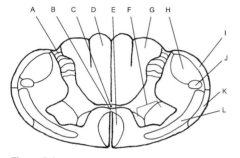

Figure 2.1

A	Dorsal horn (substantia gelatinosa)
B	Ventral white commissure
C	Central canal
D	Fasciculus gracilis
E	Ventral corticospinal tract
F	Ventral horn
G	Fasciculus cuneatus
H	Lateral corticospinal tract
I	Dorsal spinocerebellar tract
J	Rubrospinal tract
K	Ventral spinocerebellar tract
L	Spinothalamic tract

What are the connective tissue membranes that surround the central nervous system (CNS)?

Meninges

Name the three layers of meninges from outermost to innermost.

1. Dura mater
2. Arachnoid
3. Pia mater

Which layer(s) of the meninges are also known as pachymeninges, and which are known as leptomeninges?

Pachymeninges: dura mater
Leptomeninges: arachnoid and pia mater

Which meningeal space contains the cerebrospinal fluid, and at what vertebral level does this space terminate?

Subarachnoid space; S2

Which spinal nerve bundles are contained in the cauda equina?

L2-Co (coccygeal nerve)

Is the subdural space a real or potential space?	Potential space
What are the contents of the epidural space?	Adipose tissue, lymphatics, and venous plexus
At what vertebral level does the conus medullaris terminate in the adult and newborn?	L1 (adult), L3 (newborn)

Identify the spinal cord levels between which the following structures are located:

Ciliospinal center of Budge	C8-T2
Intermediolateral cell column	T1-L3
Nucleus dorsalis of Clarke (Clarke column)	C8-L2

VASCULAR SUPPLY

What is the main arterial supply of the spinal cord?	Anterior spinal artery (supplies the ventral two-thirds of the cord)
This vessel is formed from merged branches of what paired arteries?	Vertebral arteries
Which vessel(s) supply the posterior spinal cord?	Posterior spinal arteries (2)
What is the name for segmental arteries that give collateral supply to the anterior and posterior spinal arteries?	Radicular arteries
What radicular arteries are primarily responsible for supply of the thoracic, lumbar, and sacral regions of the spinal cord?	Intercostal and lumbar arteries
What two other major vessels contribute collateral supply to the caudal spinal cord?	Great anterior medullary artery of Adamkiewicz and ascending sacral artery
Occlusion of the anterior spinal artery results in characteristic sparing of which spinal tracts?	Dorsal columns

DESCENDING MOTORS TRACTS

In which spinal cord tract do the axons of upper motor neurons decussate in the caudal medulla travel?

Lateral corticospinal tract

Where does this tract lie within the spinal cord?

Dorsolaterally within the lateral column (funiculus)

What other descending motor tract travels in the lateral column spinal cord?

Rubrospinal tract

In which spinal cord tract do the nondecussating axons of upper motor neurons travel?

Ventral corticospinal tract

Where does this tract lie within the spinal cord?

Ventromedially within the ventral column

Where are the cell bodies of lower motor neurons located in the spinal cord?

Ventral horn (often referred to as anterior horn cells)

Describe the location of motor neurons for flexor muscles relative to motor neurons for extensor muscles.

Flexor motor neurons lie dorsal to extensor motor neurons within the ventral horn.

Describe the location of motor neurons for distal muscles relative to motor neurons for proximal muscles within the ventral horn.

Motor neurons of limb muscles lie lateral to motor neurons of axial muscles.

Identify the spinal cord level of the following clinically important reflex arcs:

Ankle jerk reflex	S1
Knee jerk reflex	L2-L4
Biceps jerk reflex	C5-C6
Triceps jerk reflex	C7-C8

SENSORY TRACTS

What somatosensory information is transmitted in the dorsal column—medial lemniscal system?

Conscious proprioception, vibration sense, and two-point discrimination

Which receptors supply sensory information to the dorsal column—medial lemniscal system?	Pacinian corpuscles, Meissner corpuscles, Merkel disks, Ruffini endings, muscle spindles, and Golgi tendon organs
What somatosensory information in the dorsal column—medial lemniscal system is supplied by the muscle spindle and Golgi tendon organ?	Proprioception
Where are the cell bodies of primary neurons of the dorsal column—medial lemniscal system located?	Dorsal root ganglion
Where do the primary neurons of the dorsal column—medial lemniscal system terminate?	Ipsilateral cuneate and gracile nuclei (caudal medulla)
Where are the cell bodies of secondary neurons of the dorsal column—medial lemniscal system located?	Cuneate/gracile nuclei (caudal medulla)
Where is the decussation of the dorsal column—medial lemniscal system?	Axons from the cuneate and gracile nuclei decussate as internal arcuate fibers, eventually forming the medial lemniscus.
Somatosensory information from the lower extremities travels along which axon bundle in the dorsal columns?	Gracile fasciculus
Somatosensory information from the upper extremities travels along which axon bundle in the dorsal columns?	Cuneate fasciculus
Information from which spinal levels travels in the cuneate fasciculus?	T6 and above
Describe the somatotopic organization of the dorsal columns.	Caudal nerve roots contribute to medial fibers of the dorsal columns. Rostral nerve roots contribute to lateral fibers.
Will a unilateral lesion of the dorsal column—medial lemniscal system below the level of the medial lemniscus result in contralateral or ipsilateral loss of somatosensory information?	Ipsilateral loss of somatosensory information

Where would you expect somatosensory loss from a lesion of the left gracile fasciculus?	Left lower extremity
Where would you expect somatosensory loss from a lesion of the right medial lemniscus?	Left upper and lower extremities
Integrity of which ascending spinal tract is tested by asking the patient to stand with eyes closed (Romberg sign)?	Dorsal columns
What somatosensory information travels in the anterolateral system?	Pain and temperature
Which tract is responsible for getting pain and temperature information to the primary somatosensory cortex?	Spinothalamic
Which epidermal receptors mediate somatosensory information to the anterolateral system?	Free nerve endings
Where are the cell bodies of primary afferent neurons of the anterolateral system located?	Dorsal root ganglion
Upon entering the spinal cord, where do axons of primary neurons in the anterolateral system travel?	Lissauer tract
Where are the cell bodies of secondary neurons of the anterolateral system located?	Ipsilateral dorsal horn
Where do axons of the anterolateral system decussate in the spinal cord?	Ventral white commissure
After decussating, where do axons from secondary neurons of the anterolateral system travel?	Contralateral spinal cord as the spinothalamic, and spinoreticular, spinomesencephalic tracts
Which deficit in pain and temperature sensation results from spinal cord hemisection?	Partial ipsilateral loss of pain and temperature at the level of the lesion. Complete contralateral loss of pain and temperature two segments below the lesion.

Which tract accounts for the pattern of ipsilateral pain and temperature sensory loss following hemisection?

Lissauer tract sends pain and temperature information one or two levels above and below the site of termination of primary neurons.

Describe the somatotopic organization of the spinothalamic system.

Caudal nerve afferents are found lateral and rostral afferents medial.

What somatosensory information is transmitted in the spinocerebellar and cuneocerebellar tracts?

Unconscious proprioception

Which sensory afferents and receptors supply sensory information to the spinocerebellar/cuneocerebellar tracts?

Ia and II (muscle spindle), II (Golgi tendon organ)

Where are the cell bodies of primary sensory neurons of the spinocerebellar/ cuneocerebellar tracts located?

Dorsal root ganglion

In which nucleus are the cells that form the dorsal spinocerebellar tract found?

Clarke column (ipsilateral spinal cord segments C8-L2)

Where do axons carrying unconscious proprioceptive information rostral to C8 terminate?

Accessory cuneate nucleus (ipsilateral)

What is the name given to the tract formed by axons arising from the accessory cuneate nucleus?

Cuneocerebellar tract

Where do axons of the spinocerebellar and cuneocerebellar tracts terminate?

Ipsilateral cerebellum

What is believed to be the function of the ventral spinocerebellar tract?

Feedback about improper limb movements

What is different about the trajectory of the ventral spinocerebellar tract?

While the dorsal spinocerebellar tract is uncrossed, the ventral spinocerebellar tract decussates in the spinal cord and enters the cerebellum via the superior cerebellar peduncle.

How do axons of the ventral spinocerebellar tract terminate in the ipsilateral cerebellum?

The tract crosses again in the cerebellum before reaching its final destination.

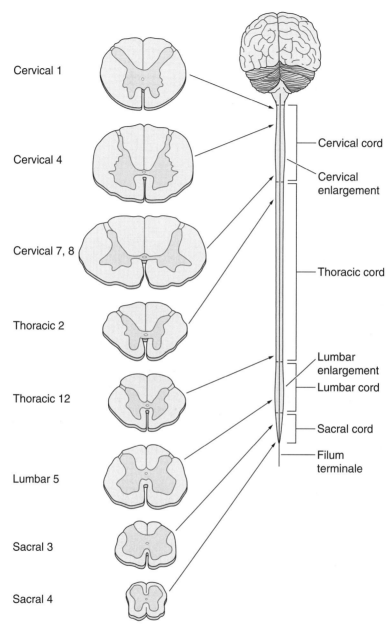

Figure 2.2   Internal and external appearances of the spinal cord at different levels. (Reproduced with permission from Kandel ER, Schwartz JH, Jessel TM, eds. *Principles of Neural Science.* 4th ed. New York, NY: McGraw-Hill; 2000: 339 .)

Which region of the spinal cord has the highest gray-to-white matter ratio?	Sacral region
Which two regions of the spinal cord contain enlargements for afferent and efferent projections of the extremities?	Cervical and lumbar
What fasciculus is present only at cervical and high thoracic levels (above T7) of the spinal cord?	Cuneate fasciculus

Identify these clinically important spinal cord lesions:

Bilateral loss of vibration and conscious proprioception, bilateral weakness and upper motor neuron signs caused by chronic B_{12} deficiency, with preservation of pain and temperature	Subacute combined degeneration
Ipsilateral loss of vibration and proprioception, ipsilateral spastic paresis, contralateral loss of pain/temperature below lesion, ipsilateral loss of pain and temperature at the level of lesion	Spinal cord hemisection (Brown-Séquard syndrome)
Bilateral spastic paresis below lesion, bilateral flaccid paresis at the level of lesion, bilateral loss of pain and temperature, with intact discriminative touch, vibration, and proprioception	Anterior spinal artery occlusion
Bilateral loss of pain and temperature across neck and shoulders, flaccid paralysis of intrinsic muscles of the hands caused by cavitation of the central canal	Syringomyelia
Bilateral loss of vibration and proprioception in patient with untreated syphilis	Tabes dorsalis (neurosyphilis)
Bilateral weakness and atrophy without sensory deficit	Amyotrophic lateral sclerosis (ALS or Lou Gehrig disease)
Random and asymmetric white matter lesions with mixed sensory and motor deficits	Multiple sclerosis

What other syndrome is included in the Brown-Séquard picture if the lesion occurs above the level of T2?	Horner syndrome
What affected spinal areas are associated with the symptoms of syringomyelia?	1. Ventral white commissure (anterolateral system) 2. Ventral horn
Which congenital malformation with cerebellar herniation is associated with syringomyelia?	Arnold-Chiari malformation

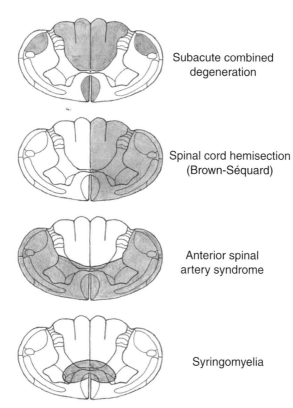

Subacute combined degeneration

Spinal cord hemisection (Brown-Séquard)

Anterior spinal artery syndrome

Syringomyelia

Figure 2.3   Anatomical depiction of common spinal cord lesion syndromes.

CLINICAL VIGNETTES

Make the diagnosis for the following patients:

A 56-year-old man who recently underwent gastric bypass surgery 8 months ago presents with weakness, skin pallor, and confusion. A neurologic test reveals decreased position and vibration sense, lower extremity ataxia with a positive bilateral Babinski reflex, and positive Romberg sign. Complete blood count (CBC) reveals a mean corpuscular volume (MCV) of 110, decreased reticulocyte count, and hypersegmented neutrophils on peripheral blood smear. Serum homocysteine and methylmalonic acid levels are elevated.

Vitamin B_{12} deficiency (subacute combined degeneration)

A 78-year-old female with no past medical history (PMH) seen for her annual physical examination complains of progressive lower back pain radiating to her legs, weakness while getting up from a sitting position, and numbness/tingling involving the buttocks and area between her thighs in a saddle-like distribution. On further questioning, patient admits to urinary incontinence. Physical examination reveals diminished reflexes in the lower extremities. MRI reveals spinal stenosis.

Cauda equina syndrome

A 28-year-old male is seen in the ER after burning his hands while cooking. Further evaluation reveals symptoms of progressive fine motor loss in his hands bilaterally. On physical examination, patient is found to have decreased pain and temperature sensation on his shoulders bilaterally in a cape-like distribution. He denies any recent trauma or medical illness, but says that he was seen 5 years ago after sustaining minor injuries in a motor vehicle accident. Initial lab studies are all within normal limits (WNL), and results from MRI of patient's cervical and thoracic spine show cystic formation and cavitation of the central canal.

Syringomyelia

A 32-year-old female presents with recent onset of pain in her right eye with progressing visual loss. Her gait is found to be unsteady and she is unable to stand without closing her eyes and supporting herself. On further questioning, the patient is found to have double vision. Physical examination is remarkable for loss of vision in patient's right upper quadrant, decreased deep tendon reflexes in her right lower extremity, and loss of proprioception in patient's lower extremities bilaterally. Lab studies are noncontributory and MRI of patient's head demonstrates diffuse white matter lesions.

Multiple sclerosis

A 42-year-old male is brought to the ER after sustaining traumatic injury in a motor vehicle accident. On physical examination, patient is found to have decreased two-point discrimination, vibration, and proprioception on the left side below the umbilicus, and loss of pain and temperature sense on the right side two levels below the umbilicus. Patient is also found unable to move his left lower extremity and general paresis is noted on the lower left side of patient's body.

Brown-Séquard syndrome T10 level on the left side

CHAPTER 3

Brainstem and Cranial Nerves

Table 3.1 Classes of Innervation

Classification	Innervation
General somatic efferent (GSE)	Skeletal muscle
General somatic afferent (GSA)	Somatosensory
General visceral efferent (GVE)	Autonomic
General visceral afferent (GVA)	Visceral sensation
Special visceral efferent (SVE)	Branchial arches
Special visceral afferent (SVA)	Taste and smell
Special somatic afferent (SSA)	Vision, audition, vestibular

From what embryologic structures do the following divisions derive:	
GSE, SVE, GVE	Basal plate
GVA, SVA, GSA, SSA	Alar plate
What is the groove that separates the alar plate from the basal plate?	Sulcus limitans
How are the alar and basal plates functionally distinct?	Alar: sensory (afferent) Basal: motor (efferent)
How are the alar and basal plates positioned anatomically in the brainstem?	Alar is dorsolateral and basal is ventromedial.

MEDULLA

Identify the labeled structures in Fig. 3.1:

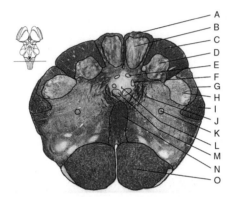

Figure 3.1   Transverse section of the caudal medulla. (Adapted with permission from Martin JH, ed. *Neuroanatomy: Text and Atlas.* 3rd ed. New York, NY: McGraw-Hill; 2003: 438.)

A	Fasciculus gracilis	I	Dorsal spinocerebellar tract
B	Nucleus gracilis	J	Internal arcuate fibers
C	Fasciculus cuneatus	K	Nucleus ambiguus
D	Nucleus cuneatus	L	Central canal
E	Solitary nucleus	M	Hypoglossal nucleus
F	Dorsal motor nucleus of X	N	Medial lemniscus
G	Spinal trigeminal tract	O	Medullary pyramid
H	Spinal trigeminal nucleus		

Identify the labeled structures in Fig. 3.2:

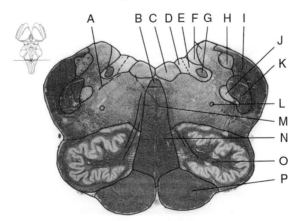

Figure 3.2   Transverse section of the rostral medulla. (Adapted with permission from Martin JH, ed. *Neuroanatomy: Text and Atlas.* 3rd ed. New York, NY: McGraw-Hill; 2003: 440.)

A	Vagus nerve fiber	I	Inferior cerebellar peduncle
B	Medial longitudinal fasciculus	J	Spinal trigeminal nucleus
C	Hypoglossal nucleus	K	Spinal trigeminal tract
D	Dorsal motor nucleus of X	L	Nucleus ambiguus
E	Solitary nucleus	M	Hypoglossal nerve fibers
F	Vestibular nuclei	N	Medial lemniscus
G	Solitary tract	O	Inferior olivary nucleus
H	Accessory cuneate nucleus	P	Medullary pyramid

Identify the labeled structures in Fig. 3.3:

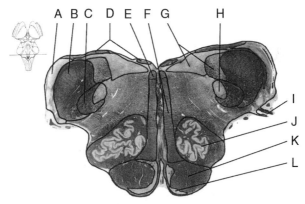

Figure 3.3   Transverse section of the rostral pons. (Adapted with permission from Martin JH, ed. *Neuroanatomy: Text and Atlas*. 3rd ed. New York, NY: McGraw-Hill; 2003: 442.)

A	Cochlear nuclei	H	Spinal trigeminal nucleus
B	Inferior cerebellar peduncle	I	Glossopharyngeal nerve fibers
C	Spinal trigeminal tract		
D	Striae medullaris	J	Inferior olivary nucleus
E	Medial longitudinal fasciculus	K	Medullary pyramid
F	Medial lemniscus	L	Arcuate nucleus
G	Vestibular nuclei		

Table 3.2 Nuclei of the Medulla[*]

Innervation	Nucleus	Function
SSA	Medial and inferior vestibular	Vestibular/balance
GSA	Spinal trigeminal nucleus	Pain and temperature; sensation of external ear from CN V, VII, IX, and X
SVA	Caudal solitary nucleus	Taste from CN IX and X
GVA	Solitary nucleus	Visceral sensation via CN IX and X
GVE	Dorsal motor nucleus of X	Parasympathetic of viscera (CN X)
	Inferior salivatory	Parasympathetic to parotid gland (CN IX)
SVE	Nucleus ambiguus	Branchial arches: 3rd via CN IX—stylopharyngeus 4th and 6th via CN X and XI—constrictors, cricothyroid, and levator veli palatini
GSE	Hypoglossal	Intrinsic tongue muscles via CN XII

[*]Note the dorsolateral to ventromedial order of nuclei.

What is the large and vaguely defined group of nuclei extending from caudal medulla to the diencephalon?	Reticular formation
In what processes is the reticular formation involved?	Arousal, autonomic function, reflexes, and behavior
Which ascending spinal tract transmits information about tactile discrimination, proprioception, and vibration sense?	Dorsal columns
What nuclei contain second order neurons of the dorsal column medial–lemniscal system?	Nucleus gracilis (legs) and nucleus cuneatus (arms)
Where is the decussation of the dorsal column–medial lemniscus system?	Internal arcuate fibers in the caudal medulla

In what tract do axons of the dorsal column–medial lemniscus system ascend to the thalamus after decussating?	Medial lemniscus
What thalamic nucleus contains third order neurons of the dorsal column–medial lemniscus system?	Ventral posterolateral nucleus (VPL)
What spinal tract transmits pain and temperature information from the contralateral side of the body?	Spinothalamic tract (anterolateral system)
Where are the first-order neurons of the anterolateral system?	Dorsal root ganglion (DRG)
Where are the second-order neurons of the anterolateral system?	Ipsilateral dorsal horn of the spinal cord
Where does the lateral spinothalamic tract decussate?	Ventral white commissure of spinal cord
In which thalamic nucleus does the spinothalamic tract terminate?	VPL
What tract carries pain and temperature information from the trigeminal nerve, as well as sensory information from the external ear from CN VII, IX, and X?	Spinal trigeminal tract
Where are the second-order neurons of the spinal trigeminal system located?	Ipsilateral spinal trigeminal nucleus
Describe the course of axons from second-order neurons of the spinal trigeminal tract:	Axons from the spinal trigeminal nucleus decussate and ascend as the contralateral ventral trigeminothalamic tract terminating in the thalamus.
In which thalamic nucleus does the ventral trigeminothalamic tract terminate?	Ventral posteromedial nucleus (VPM)
Where are fibers of the corticospinal tract located in the medulla?	Medullary pyramids
At what level do the descending fibers of the corticospinal tract decussate?	Medulla-spinal cord junction

Second-order neurons of which tract originate in the accessory cuneate nucleus?	Cuneocerebellar tract
What is the function of the cuneocerebellar tract?	Transmits unconscious proprioceptive information from the upper limbs to cerebellum
What tract transmits proprioceptive information from the lower limbs to the cerebellum?	Dorsal spinocerebellar tract
What spinal nucleus is analogous to the accessory cuneate nucleus and extends from C8 to L2?	Nucleus dorsalis of Clarke
Which cerebellar peduncle transmits the dorsal spinocerebellar and cuneocerebellar tracts to the cerebellum?	Inferior cerebellar peduncle
To which descending motor pathways do efferents from the inferior cerebellar peduncle contribute?	Vestibulospinal and reticulospinal tracts
Which proprioceptive tract enters the cerebellum via the superior cerebellar peduncle?	Ventral spinocerebellar tract
What tract extends from the mesencephalon to the medulla and conveys information from the red nucleus to the inferior olivary nucleus?	Central tegmental tract
What are the excitatory fibers that project from the inferior olivary nucleus to the cerebellum called?	Climbing fibers
What are the other major excitatory input fibers into the cerebellum?	Mossy fibers
Axons of which other neurons are contained within the central tegmental tract?	Second-order taste neurons (SVA) projecting from the rostral solitary nucleus, viscerosensory neurons (GVA) projecting to the parabrachial nucleus of the pons and posteromedial nucleus of the thalamus

PONS

Identify the labeled structures in Fig. 3.4:

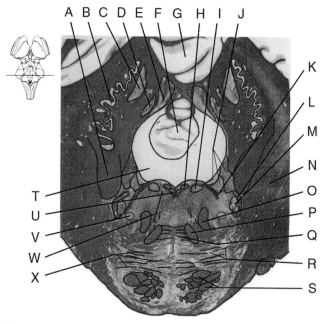

Figure 3.4 Transverse section of the mid-pons. (Adapted with permission from Martin JH, ed. *Neuroanatomy: Text and Atlas.* 3rd ed. New York, NY: McGraw-Hill; 2003: 444.)

A	Superior cerebellar peduncle		N	Middle cerebellar peduncle
B	Dentate nucleus		O	Central tegmental tract
C	Emboliform nucleus		P	Medial lemniscus
D	Globose nucleus		Q	Trapezoid body
E	Fastigial nucleus		R	Pontine nuclei
F	Nodulus		S	Corticospinal and corticobulbar tracts
G	Cerebellar vermis			
H	Genu of facial nerve		T	Fourth ventricle
I	Abducens nucleus		U	Medial longitudinal fasciculus
J	Vestibular nuclei		V	Facial nucleus
K	Facial nerve fibers		W	Abducens nerve fibers
L	Spinal trigeminal tract		X	Pontocerebellar fibers
M	Spinal trigeminal nucleus			

Identify the labeled structures in Fig. 3.5:

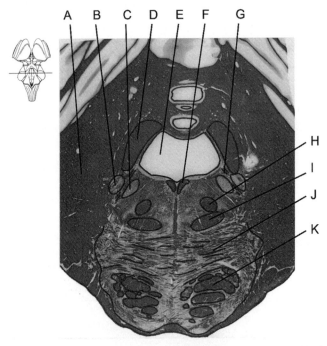

Figure 3.5   Transverse section of the rostral pons. (Adapted with permission from Martin JH, ed. *Neuroanatomy: Text and Atlas.* 3rd ed. New York, NY: McGraw-Hill; 2003: 446.)

A	Middle cerebellar peduncle	G	Trigeminal nerve fibers
B	Principle trigeminal sensory nucleus	H	Central tegmental tract
		I	Medial lemniscus
C	Trigeminal motor nucleus	J	Pontocerebellar fibers
D	Superior cerebellar peduncle	K	Corticospinal and corticobulbar tracts
E	Fourth ventricle		
F	Medial longitudinal fasciculus		

Table 3.3 Pontine Nuclei

Innervation	Nucleus	Function
SSA	Medial, lateral, and superior vestibular	Vestibular/balance/eye movements
GSA	Principal sensory nucleus of CN V	Vibration, discriminative touch, and pressure for face
SVA	Rostral solitary nucleus	Taste from CN VII
GVA	—	—
GVE	Superior salivatory	Parasympathetic of lacrimal, sublingual, and submandibular gland (CN VII)
SVE		Branchial arches:
	Motor nucleus of CN V	First arch—muscles of mastication
	Motor nucleus of CN VII	Second arch—muscles of facial expression and stapedius
GSE	Motor nucleus of CN VI	Innervate lateral rectus

What descending motor pathways course through the base of the pons?	Corticobulbar, corticospinal, and corticopontine tracts
What is the function of the corticobulbar tract?	Motor innervation to all motor cranial nerve nuclei (except nuclei involved in extraocular movements)
Are projections of the corticobulbar tract bilateral or unilateral?	Mostly bilateral
Which cranial nerve nuclei do not receive bilateral corticobulbar input?	Lower division of CNVII (contralateral input) (sometimes hypoglossal)
What deficit in facial movement is associated with unilateral damage to the corticobulbar tract?	Inability to move the contralateral lower facial muscles, with sparing of muscles overlying the forehead
What deficit in facial movement is associated with unilateral damage to the facial nerve (Bell palsy/peripheral VII)?	Inability to move all ipsilateral facial muscles, including muscles of the forehead

What clinical test is used to determine whether the lesion is central or peripheral?	Eyebrow raise (upper division) Smile (lower division)
Which cerebellar peduncle carries fibers from pontine nuclei to the cerebellum?	Middle cerebellar peduncle
What tract provides the major input to the pontine nuclei?	Corticopontine tract
What is the function of the corticopontine tract?	Communicate motor information from cortex to cerebellum
What nucleus receives discriminatory touch, pressure, and vibration inputs from the face?	Principal sensory nucleus of CN V
Where do second-order neurons arising in the principal sensory nucleus of CN V project?	Contralateral ventral posterior medial nucleus of the thalamus (VPM)
Within the pontine segment of the medial lemniscus, where are fibers innervating the arms and legs found, respectively?	Arms are medial, legs are lateral.
What is the white matter tract extending through the brainstem that contains fibers from vestibular nuclei and extraocular motor nuclei?	Medial longitudinal fasciculus (MLF)
What pontine structure controls lateral gaze?	Paramedian pontine reticular formation (PPRF)
Describe how PPRF controls lateral conjugate gaze to the right:	Axons project from the right PPRF to the ipsilateral abducens nucleus. Two types of neurons found in the abducens nucleus are stimulated: (1) neurons that stimulate the right lateral rectus muscle, and (2) neurons that decussate and project through the contralateral MLF to the left oculomotor nucleus. Projections to the left oculomotor nucleus stimulate left medial rectus.

What deficit is associated with abducens nerve palsy?	Medial deviation of the ipsilateral eye due to lateral rectus paralysis
What deficit is associated with abducens nucleus injury?	Lateral gaze palsy: inability to gaze to the side of the lesion with either eye
What accounts for the difference between abducens nucleus and nerve lesions?	Nucleus injury interrupts both ipsilateral and contralateral projections (to oculomotor nucleus), whereas nerve injury only interrupts innervation of the ipsilateral lateral rectus muscle.
What is the name given to a lesion of the MLF?	Internuclear ophthalmoplegia
What is the most common cause of internuclear ophthalmoplegia?	Multiple sclerosis
What extraocular deficit is associated with internuclear ophthalmoplegia?	The eye ipsilateral to the lesion does not adduct, and the contralateral eye exhibits nystagmus.
How can clinicians verify that the medial rectus is not paralyzed in cases of internuclear ophthalmoplegia or abducens nucleus injury causing lateral gaze palsy?	Convergence is intact.
What brainstem center controls vertical gaze control?	riMLF (rostral interstitial nucleus of the medial longitudinal fasciculus)
What syndrome causes upward gaze palsy by compressing the dorsal midbrain?	Parinaud syndrome
Which cortical centers control saccadic eye movements to the contralateral side?	Frontal eye fields (FEF)
Unilateral FEF lesions cause deviation of the eyes to which side?	Ipsilateral

MESENCEPHALON

Identify the labeled structures in Fig. 3.6:

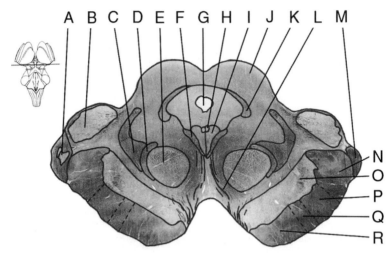

Figure 3.6 Transverse section of the rostral midbrain. (Adapted with permission from Martin JH, ed. *Neuroanatomy: Text and Atlas.* 3rd ed. New York, NY: McGraw-Hill; 2003: 452.)

A	Lateral geniculate nucleus	L	Oculomotor nerve fibers
B	Medial geniculate nucleus	M	Optic tract
C	Medial lemniscus	N	Corticopontine tract
D	Cerebellothalamic fibers		(parietal/temporal/occipital)
E	Red nucleus	O	Substantia nigra
F	Interstitial nucleus of MLF	P	Corticospinal tract
G	Cerebral aqueduct	Q	Corticobulbar tract
H	Edinger-Westphal nucleus	R	Corticopontine tract (frontal)
I	Oculomotor nucleus		
J	Superior colliculus		
K	Mesencephalic trigeminal nucleus		

Table 3.4 Midbrain Nuclei

Innervation	Nucleus	Function
SSA	—	—
GSA	Mesencephalic nucleus of CN V	Proprioception of jaw and extraocular muscles (jaw jerk reflex)
SVA	—	—
GVA	—	—
GVE	Edinger-Westphal (E-W)	Pupilloconstrictor reflex and accommodation
SVE	—	—
GSE	Motor nucleus of CN III	Innervates extraoculars except LR and SO
	Motor nucleus of CN IV	Innervates the superior oblique

Abbreviations: LR, lateral rectus and SO, superior oblique.

What is the tectum?	The roof of the midbrain, defined as all structures dorsal to the cerebral aqueduct, including the superior and inferior colliculi
What is the tegmentum?	Region of the midbrain between the cerebral aqueduct and the basis pedunculi
What is the basis pedunculi?	Also called the crus cerebri, it is the "legs" that carry the corticobulbar, corticospinal, corticopontine tracts, in addition to the substantia nigra.
What are the cerebral peduncles?	Combination of the tegmentum and the basis pedunculi
What structure connects the third and fourth ventricles?	Cerebral aqueduct (of Sylvius)
What structure surrounds the cerebral aqueduct?	Periaqueductal gray

What is the function of the periaqueductal gray?	Endogenous pain suppression
What is the function of the locus coeruleus?	Provides diffuse norepinephrine projections in the CNS
Name the two divisions of the substantia nigra.	1. Pars reticularis 2. Pars compacta
Which division contains dopaminergic neurons?	Pars compacta (pars reticularis contains GABAergic neurons)
Where does the pars compacta project?	Through the nigrostriatal tract to the striatum (caudate/putamen)
What disease is associated with loss of pars compacta neurons?	Parkinson disease
Where does the pars reticularis project?	Thalamus, pedunculopontine nucleus, and the superior colliculus (plays a role in controlling saccadic eye movement)
What is the ventral midbrain structure that contains dopaminergic neurons that project to the striatum and to the prefrontal cortex?	Ventral tegmental area
What structure receives visual input directly from the retina, occipital lobes, and FEFs and mediates audiovisual reflexes, searching, and tracking?	Superior colliculus
Name the nucleus that receives visual input from retinal ganglion cells and projects bilaterally to the E-W nuclei, mediating the pupillary light reflex.	Pretectal nucleus
Across what commissure does input to the contralateral E-W nucleus travel?	Posterior commissure
What is the only cranial nerve that crosses the midline?	CN IV (trochlear)
Why is this important?	All other cranial nerve injuries result in ipsilateral defects.
What nucleus at the level of the superior colliculus mediates flexor tone?	Red nucleus
In what tract do rubro-olivary fibers travel?	Central tegmental tract

Through which cerebellar peduncle do cerebellar efferents enter the midbrain?

Superior cerebellar peduncle

At what level do the superior cerebellar peduncles decussate?

In the midbrain at the level of the inferior colliculi

BRAINSTEM LESIONS

Occlusion of branches of what artery causes medial medullary syndrome?

Vertebral artery or the caudal aspect of the basilar artery

What structures are often injured in medial medullary syndrome?

Hypoglossal nerve, pyramidal tract, and medial lemniscus

What are the symptoms of medial medullary syndrome?

Ipsilateral paralysis of tongue, contralateral paralysis of arm and leg (spares face), and contralateral loss of discriminative touch, vibration, and proprioception

Occlusion of what artery causes lateral medullary (Wallenberg) syndrome?

Vertebral, posterior inferior cerebellar artery (PICA), or any of the lateral medullary arteries

What structures are typically injured in lateral medullary syndrome?

Medial and inferior vestibular nuclei, inferior cerebellar peduncle, nucleus ambiguus, glossopharyngeal and vagus nerve, spinothalamic tract, spinal trigeminal tract and/or nucleus, descending sympathetic fibers, nucleus gracilis and cuneatus, and sometimes solitary tract/nucleus

What are the symptoms of lateral medullary syndrome?

Ipsilateral: numbness/pain over half of face, numbness of arms, leg, and trunk, ataxia/falling to the side of the lesion, dysphagia, paralysis of vocal cord, ↓ gag reflex, paralysis of palate, loss of taste, nystagmus, diplopia, oscillopsia, vertigo, nausea, vomiting, and Horner syndrome (ptosis, miosis, anhydrosis)

Contralateral: impaired pain and thermal sense over half the body

What are the symptoms of locked-in syndrome?

Nearly all motor pathways are lesioned, leaving only extraocular muscle innervation intact. Patients have paralysis of the body and facial muscles.

What is an iatrogenic cause of locked-in syndrome?

Central pontine myelinolysis—caused by correcting hyponatremia too quickly

What tracts are injured in locked-in syndrome?

Bilateral corticobulbar and corticospinal tracts

Where is the typical location of this lesion?

Base of the pons

What causes dorsal midbrain (Parinaud) syndrome?

Damage to the posterior commissure, superior colliculus, and pretectal nucleus usually due to a pineal tumor compressing the tectum

What are the symptoms of dorsal midbrain (Parinaud) syndrome?

Vertical gaze palsy, with nystagmus on attempted vertical gaze, and loss of pupillary reflex

Occlusion of what vessel(s) causes Benedikt syndrome?

Paramedian arteries of the posterior cerebral artery

What structures are injured in Benedikt syndrome?

Oculomotor nerve, red nucleus, and medial lemniscus

What are the symptoms of Benedikt syndrome?

Ipsilateral oculomotor palsy causing the classic "down and out" appearance with ptosis and fixed pupillary dilation, cerebellar dystaxia with intention tremor, contralateral loss of discriminative touch, vibration, and proprioception

Benedikt syndrome is caused by occlusion of what vessels?

Branches of the basilar and posterior cerebral arteries

What structures are injured in Weber syndrome?

Oculomotor nerve and cerebral peduncle

What are the symptoms of Weber syndrome?

Ipsilateral third nerve palsy (down and out, fixed pupil dilation, ptosis), diplopia, and contralateral hemiplegia

Weber syndrome is caused by occlusion of what vessels?

Short paramedian branches of the basilar and posterior cerebral arteries (see Chap. 9)

Table 3.5 Brainstem Syndromes: Symptoms and the Structures Responsible*

Syndrome	Affected Structure	Symptom
Medial medullary syndrome	Medial lemniscus	Contra. loss of vibration and proprioception
	Medullary pyramid	Contra. limb paralysis
	Hypoglossal nerve and nucleus	Deviation of tongue to ipsi side
Lateral medullary syndrome	Vestibular nuclei	Nystagmus, diplopia, vertigo, nausea
	Inferior cerebellar peduncle	Ipsilateral ataxia/falling
	Nucleus ambiguus	Hoarseness, dysphagia
	CN IX and X	Dysphagia/gag reflex
	Spinothalamic tract	Contra. loss of body pain/temp
	Spinal trigeminal tract/nucleus	Ipsi. loss of face pain/temp
	Descending sympathetics	Horner syndrome
	Nucleus gracilis/cuneatus	Ipsilateral body numbness
	Solitary tract/nucleus	Loss of tastes
Locked-in syndrome	Corticobulbar tract	Bilateral facial paralysis
	Corticospinal tract	Bilateral limb and torso paralysis
Benedikt syndrome	Oculomotor nerve (CN III)	Ipsi. "down and out" eye, ptosis, fixed pupil dilation, diplopia
	Red nucleus	Involuntary movements/chorea and tremor
	Medial lemniscus	Contra. loss of touch, vibration, proprioception
	Cerebellothalamic fibers	Contra. ataxia/intention tremor
Weber syndrome	Oculomotor nerve (CN III)	Ipsi "down and out" eye, ptosis, fixed pupil dilation, diplopia
	Cerebral peduncle	Contra. spastic hemiplegia

Abbreviations: contra, contralateral and ipsi, ipsilateral.
*Also see Fig. 3.7.

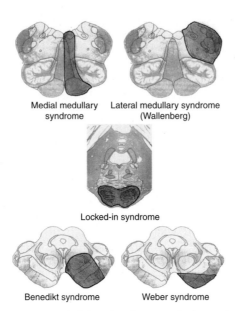

Figure 3.7   Anatomical depiction of common brainstem lesions.

CRANIAL NERVES

Identify the labeled structures in Fig. 3.8.

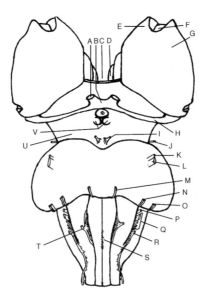

Figure 3.8   Anatomic diagram of the ventral brainstem. (Adapted with permission from Martin JH, ed. *Neuroanatomy: Text and Atlas.* 3rd ed. New York, NY: McGraw-Hill; 2003: 418.)

A	Optic nerve	L	Sensory root of trigeminal nerve
B	Optic chiasm	M	Abducens nerve
C	Third ventricle	N	Facial nerve
D	Thalamus	O	Vestibulocochlear nerve
E	Head of caudate	P	Glossopharyngeal nerve
F	Internal capsule	Q	Vagus nerve
G	Putamen	R	Spinal accessory nerve
H	Optic tract	S	Pyramidal decussation
I	Oculomotor nerve	T	Hypoglossal nerve
J	Trochlear nerve	U	Cerebral peduncle
K	Motor root of trigeminal nerve	V	Mammillary bodies

Which is the only cranial nerve that exits the brainstem from the dorsal surface?	CN IV (trochlear)
Which cranial nerves exit the midbrain?	CN III (oculomotor) and CN IV (trochlear)
Which cranial nerves exit at the level of the pons?	Midpons: CN V (trigeminal) Pontomedullary junction: CN VI (abducens) CN VII (facial) CN VIII (vestibulocochlear)
Which cranial nerves exit at the level of the medulla?	CN IX (glossopharyngeal), CN X (vagus), CN XI (spinal accessory), and CN XII (hypoglossal)
Which cranial nerves are sensory, motor, and mixed?	Sensory: I, II, VIII Motor: III, IV, VI, XI, XII Mixed: V, VII, IX, X

Identify the labeled structures in Fig. 3.9.

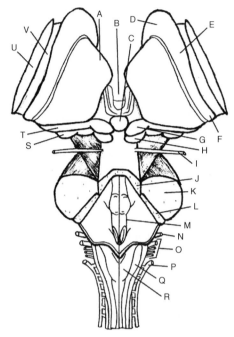

Figure 3.9   Anatomic diagram of the dorsal brainstem. (Adapted with permission from Martin JH, ed. *Neuroanatomy: Text and Atlas.* 3rd ed. New York, NY: McGraw-Hill; 2003:.422.)

A	Thalamus	L	Inferior cerebellar peduncle
B	Third ventricle	M	Sulcus limitans
C	Pineal gland	N	Glossopharyngeal nerve
D	Head of caudate	O	Vagus nerve
E	Body of caudate	P	Spinal accessory nerve
F	Tail of caudate	Q	Cuneate tubercle
G	Superior colliculus	R	Gracile tubercle
H	Inferior colliculus	S	Medial geniculate body
I	Trochlear nerve	T	Lateral geniculate body
J	Superior cerebellar peduncle	U	Putamen
K	Middle cerebellar peduncle	V	Internal capsule

Name the only CNS nucleus that contains pseudounipolar primary sensory neurons of neural crest origin.

Mesencephalic trigeminal nucleus—contains cell bodies of stretch receptors found in muscles of mastication

Through what foramen does each cranial nerve pass?	I: cribriform plate
	II: optic canal
	III: superior orbital fissure
	IV: superior orbital fissure
	V1: superior orbital fissure
	V2: foramen rotundum
	V3: foramen ovale
	VI: superior orbital fissure
	VII: internal auditory meatus
	VIII: internal auditory meatus
	IX: jugular foramen
	X: jugular foramen
	XI: jugular foramen
	XII: hypoglossal canal
To what CNS nucleus does the olfactory nerve project?	Olfactory bulb
What cranial nerve is made of retinal ganglion cell axons?	CN II (optic)
Where do the axons of the retinal ganglion cells synapse?	Majority: lateral geniculate nucleus of the thalamus
	Minority: superior colliculus and pretectal nucleus
What CNS nucleus contains the motor neurons that innervate the superior rectus, inferior rectus, medial rectus, lateral rectus, inferior oblique, and levator palpebrae?	Oculomotor nucleus
What CNS nucleus contains neurons that control the ciliary muscle and sphincter muscle of the pupil?	E-W nucleus of oculomotor complex
Describe the pathway of parasympathetic fibers originating in the E-W nucleus.	1. E-W 2. Ciliary ganglion 3. Short ciliary nerve 4. Ciliary muscle/sphincter muscle
What type of injury to CN III will produce ipsilateral ptosis and extraocular muscle palsy in a "down and out" pattern, without causing a fixed dilated pupil?	Damage to the central fibers of CN III, as in diabetic ischemic neuropathy

What type of injury to CN III will produce an ipsilateral fixed dilated pupil?

Compromise of the peripheral fibers of CN III, as in compression

What are some causes of CN III compression?

Uncal (transtentorial) herniation resulting from increased intracranial pressure, aneurysm of posterior cerebral artery, and aneurysm of superior cerebellar artery

What accounts for the different physical findings associated with compression and microvascular injury of CN III?

Parasympathetic fibers travel on the periphery of CN III, and are the first to be damaged by a compression injury. Motor fibers are located deep in the nerve, and are the most vulnerable to ischemic injury that occurs in diabetic neuropathy.

What muscle does CN IV (trochlear) innervate?

Superior oblique

What is the action of the superior oblique?

Turns eyeball inferomedially (intorts)

What is the classic symptom associated with trochlear nerve palsy?

Diplopia when looking down (going down stairs/reading)

How do patients compensate for trochlear nerve palsy?

Incline the head anteriorly and toward the side of the normal eye

What muscles do V1 (ophthalmic), V2 (maxillary), and V3 (mandibular) trigeminal nerve divisions innervate?

V1 and V2 do not innervate any muscles. V3 innervates muscles of mastication (temporalis, masseter, lateral pterygoid, medial pterygoid), tensor tympani, tensor palati, and anterior belly of digastric.

From what branchial arch are these muscles derived?

First branchial arch

What nerve innervates lateral rectus muscle?

CN VI (abducens)

What is the appearance of the eye in CN VI palsy?

Medial deviation of the ipsilateral eye

What are some causes of CN VI injury?

Compression due to increased intracranial pressure or space-occupying lesion, cavernous sinus thrombosis, and impingement by an atherosclerotic internal carotid artery

What nerve conveys general sensory information from the tongue?	Anterior 2/3: CN V3, via lingual nerve Posterior 1/3: CN IX
What nerves convey taste?	Anterior 2/3 of tongue and palate: CN VII, via chorda tympani Posterior 1/3 of tongue: CN IX Posterior oropharynx and larynx: CN X
In what peripheral sensory ganglia are primary sensory neurons involved in taste located?	CN VII: geniculate ganglion CN IX: petrosal ganglion CN X: inferior nodose ganglion
In what CNS nucleus do primary sensory fibers involved in taste synapse?	All converge on the rostral solitary nucleus.
What do neurons of the superior salivatory nucleus innervate?	Lacrimal, submandibular, and sublingual gland
Describe the course of these axons.	Fibers travel via CN VII. Axons controlling the lacrimal gland synapse in the pterygopalatine ganglion. Axons controlling the submandibular and sublingual gland synapse in the submandibular ganglion.
What do neurons of the inferior salivatory nucleus innervate?	Parotid gland
Describe the course of these axons.	Parasympathetic fibers originate in the inferior salivatory nucleus, travel via CN IX, and synapse in the otic ganglion, which projects to the parotid gland.
What muscles are innervated by CN VII?	Muscles of facial expression, stapedius, posterior belly of digastric, and stylohyoid
From which branchial arch are these muscles derived?	Second branchial arch
What type of neuron innervates the hair cells of the cochlea?	Bipolar primary sensory neurons
What peripheral sensory ganglion contains these bipolar sensory neurons?	Spiral ganglion

In what nuclei do these bipolar sensory neurons synapse?	Ipsilateral cochlear nuclei found in the rostral medulla
What are the functional roles of the anteroventral, posteroventral, and dorsal cochlear nuclei?	Anteroventral: horizontal localization of sound Posteroventral: hair cell sensitivity Dorsal: vertical localization of sound
What muscle(s) does CN IX (glossopharyngeal) innervate?	Stylopharyngeus
From which branchial arch is this muscle derived?	Third branchial arch
What CNS nucleus contains the neurons that project through CN IX to innervate stylopharyngeus?	Nucleus ambiguus
To what nucleus do sensory fibers innervating the external ear canal project?	Spinal trigeminal nucleus
Which cranial nerves transmit the sensory fibers that innervate the external ear canal?	CN V3, VII, IX, and X
What is the function of the caudal solitary nucleus?	Relay viscerosensory information from the larynx, trachea, gut (proximal to splenic flexure), and aortic arch receptors carried by the vagus nerve
In what ganglion do you find the cell bodies of vagal neurons innervating the caudal solitary nucleus?	Inferior nodose ganglion
From what CNS nucleus do parasympathetic fibers traveling in CN X (vagus) arise?	Dorsal motor nucleus of CN X and nucleus ambiguus—innervate gut (to the splenic flexure) and the heart
From what CNS nucleus do branchiomeric motor fibers traveling in CN X (vagus) arise?	Nucleus ambiguus—innervate all muscles of larynx, all muscles of the pharynx (except stylopharyngeus), and all muscles of soft palate (except tensor palate)
From which branchial arch are these muscles derived?	Fourth branchial arch
What muscles are innervated by CN XI (spinal accessory)?	Sternocleidomastoid and trapezius

From which branchial arch are these muscles derived?

Sixth branchial arch

Name the muscles that CN XII (hypoglossal) innervates.

Hyoglossus, genioglossus, and styloglossus

What muscle with the suffix -glossus is not innervated by the hypoglossal nerve?

Palatoglossus is innervated by the vagus

Table 3.6 Cranial Nerve Reflexes and Tests

Cranial Nerve	Reflex	Clinical Exam
Olfactory (CN I)	—	Odor in single nostril
Optic (CN II)	Pupillary constriction (afferent)	Visual acuity and fields Swinging flashlight
Oculomotor (CN III)	Pupillary constriction (efferent)	Pupillary reflex Extraocular H-test
Trochlear (CN IV)	—	Extraocular H-test
Trigeminal (CN V)	Corneal (afferent) Jaw jerk (both)	Facial sensation Jaw clench
Abducens (CN VI)	—	Extraocular H-test
Facial (CN VII)	Corneal (efferent)	Wrinkle forehead and smile
Vestibulocochlear (CN VIII)	—	Gross hearing Caloric testing
Glossopharyngeal (CN IX)	Gag reflex (afferent)	Palatal elevation
Vagus (CN X)	Gag reflex (efferent)	Palatal elevation
Spinal accessory (CN IX)	—	Shoulder shrug
Hypoglossal (CN XII)	—	Tongue protrusion

Table 3.7 Signs of Cranial Nerve Injury

Injured Nerve	Abnormal Finding
Olfactory (CN I)	Anosmia—loss of olfaction
Optic (CN II)	Blindness, field abnormality Marcus Gunn pupil (loss of direct pupillary response)
Oculomotor (CN III)	Dilated pupil Loss of pupillary reflex (direct and consensual) Diplopia (double vision) Ptosis and lateral deviation of the eye
Trochlear (CN IV)	Diplopia on downgaze Head tilting on downgaze
Trigeminal (CN V)	Loss of facial sensation and/or neuralgia Weakness/asymmetry on mastication Lack of corneal reflex Lack of jaw jerk reflex
Abducens (CN VI)	Diplopia Medial deviation of affected eye Inability to abduct the affected eye
Facial (CN VII)	Weakness of muscles of facial expression (Bell palsy) Loss of corneal reflex Loss of taste (anterior 2/3 of tongue) Reduced salivation and tearing Hyperacusis (stapedius innervation)
Vestibulocochlear (CN VIII)	Hearing loss/tinnitus Vertigo Nystagmus
Glossopharyngeal (CN IX)	Loss of taste over posterior 1/3 of tongue Loss of sensation in posterior tongue and palate Loss of gag reflex Reduced salivation
Vagus (CN X)	Hoarseness Loss of gag reflex Dysphagia—difficulty in swallowing
Spinal accessory (CN IX)	Weakness and wasting of trapezius and sternocleidomastoid
Hypoglossal (CN XII)	Deviation toward affected side Wasting of tongue muscles

CLINICAL VIGNETTES

Make the diagnosis for the following patient:

A 65-year-old female with a history of atherosclerosis presents with left-sided loss of sensation on body, right-sided sensory deficit of face, and unsteadiness when walking. Physical examination is significant for sensory deficit of left side of body and right side of face, dysmetria, and ataxia. Brain imaging confirms the suspected diagnosis.

> Wallenberg syndrome (lateral medullary syndrome)

A 51-year-old female presented with diplopia, left ptosis, right hemiataxia and hyperactive tendon reflexes. Left pupil was dilated and unresponsive to light. Radiological examination revealed stenosis of the posterior cerebral artery and a left-sided midbrain infarct.

> Benedikt syndrome

A 55-year-old woman with a history of atrial fibrillation complains of diplopia. She also feels weakness in her left arm and leg. Her husband noticed that her right eyelid was drooping. On physical examination, the right eyelid did not open fully and the right eye was laterally deviated. Only the left eye constricted in response to light. She had facial weakness on the left. Motor strength was reduced on the left side of her body with normal sensation for the face and body.

> Weber syndrome

A 6-year-old boy was noticed by his mother to have signs of precocious puberty. Physical examination revealed a bilateral paralysis of upward gaze and a questionable weakness of convergence. The pupils constricted upon convergence but not in response to light. Radiographic studies revealed a pineal tumor.

> Parinaud syndrome

CHAPTER 4

Cerebral Anatomy

Identify the labeled structures in Fig. 4.1:

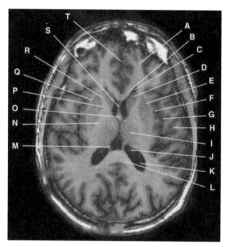

Figure 4.1 T1-weighted axial MRI section of a human brain. (*Courtesy of Michael Lipton, MD*)

A	Frontal lobe	L	Splenium of corpus callosum
B	Genu of corpus callosum	M	Crus of fornix
C	Lateral ventricle (anterior horn)	N	Posterior limb of internal capsule
D	Head of caudate nucleus		
E	Putamen	O	Body of fornix
F	Insular cortex	P	Genu of internal capsule
G	Lateral sulcus	Q	External capsule
H	Temporal lobe	R	Anterior limb of internal capsule
I	Thalamus		
J	Choroid plexus	S	Septum pellucidum
K	Lateral ventricle (atrium)	T	Sagittal fissure

Identify the labeled structures in Fig. 4.2:

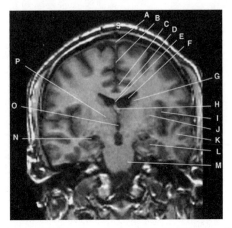

Figure 4.2   T1-weighted coronal MRI section of a human brain. (*Courtesy of Michael Lipton, MD*)

A	Superior sagittal sinus	J	Putamen
B	Falx cerebri	K	Temporal lobe
C	Cingulate gyrus	L	Hippocampus
D	Body of corpus callosum	M	Pons
E	Septum pellucidum	N	Temporal horn of lateral
F	Lateral ventricle		ventricle
G	Caudate nucleus	O	Third ventricle
H	Fornix	P	Thalamus
I	Insular cortex		

Identify the labeled structures in Fig. 4.3:

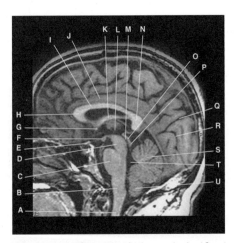

Figure 4.3   T1-weighted sagittal MRI section of a human brain. (*Courtesy of Michael Lipton, MD*)

A	Spinal cord	L	Third ventricle
B	Medulla	M	Cerebral aqueduct
C	Pons	N	Splenium of corpus callosum
D	Midbrain	O	Superior colliculus
E	Optic chiasm	P	Inferior colliculus
F	Mammillary body	Q	Parietooccipital sulcus
G	Anterior commissure	R	Calcarine fissure
H	Genu of corpus callosum	S	Vermis of cerebellum
I	Body of corpus callosum	T	Fourth ventricle
J	Cingulate gyrus	U	Nodulus of cerebellum
K	Fornix		

Table 4.1 Differences between T1- and T2 MRI Images

	T1	T2
Fat	Bright	Dark
Water	Very dark	Very bright
White matter	Bright	Dark
Gray matter	Dark	Bright
CSF	Very dark	Very bright

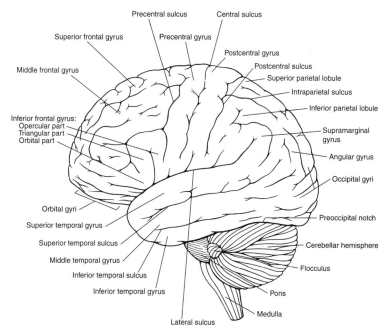

Figure 4.4 Lateral view and anatomy of the left cerebral hemisphere. (Reproduced with permission from Martin JH, ed. *Neuroanatomy: Text and Atlas.* 3rd ed. New York, NY: McGraw-Hill; 2003: 411.)

Where do the corticospinal and corticobulbar tracts primarily originate?	Precentral gyrus (or primary motor cortex)
In which lobe of the cerebral cortex is the precentral gyrus located?	Frontal lobe
Name the large pyramidal neurons of the precentral gyrus which give rise to the corticobulbar and corticospinal tracts:	Betz cells
The Betz cells are found in which cortical layer?	Layer V
Which cortical layers are strongly developed within the primary sensory cortex to receive afferent impulses?	Layers II and IV
Neurons found in layer VI of the cortex mainly project to what structure?	Thalamus
Sensory information from the ventral posterolateral (VPL) and ventral posteromedial (VPM) nuclei of the thalamus ascends to what part of the cerebral cortex?	Postcentral gyrus (or primary somatosensory cortex)
The corpus callosum lies beneath which gyrus?	Cingulate gyrus
What is the representation of the parts of the body along the sensory and motor strip of the cerebral cortex called?	Homunculus
The hypothalamus abuts which ventricle?	Third ventricle
What connects the hypothalamus to the pituitary?	Hypophyseal stalk or infundibulum
The caudate nucleus is adjacent to which ventricle?	Lateral ventricle
What sulcus or groove separates the frontal and parietal lobes?	Central sulcus
The lateral (Sylvian) fissure separates the temporal lobe from which other two lobes?	Parietal and frontal lobes

The calcarine fissure is found on the medial surface of which lobe?	Occipital lobe
The foramen of Monro connects which ventricles?	Lateral and third ventricles
From the fourth ventricle to the subarachnoid spaces, cerebrospinal fluid (CSF) flows through which foramen(a)?	Magendie (midline) and Luschka (lateral)

FRONTAL LOBE

The frontal lobe lies anterior to what sulcus?	Central (Rolandic) sulcus
The medial portion of the frontal lobe is supplied by what artery?	Anterior cerebral artery
What artery supplies the lateral portion?	Middle cerebral artery
What frontal lobe regions are associated with execution of voluntary movement?	Primary motor, premotor, and supplementary motor areas
Which frontal lobe region is responsible for social context and executive function?	Prefrontal area
What are the "executive functions" of the prefrontal cortex?	Planning, judgment, mental flexibility, abstract thinking, and working memory
What is working memory?	Type of memory used to store data for immediate mental processing and manipulation
Which region of the prefrontal cortex is associated with executive function?	Dorsolateral prefrontal cortex
What kind of manifestations might be expected with a lesion in this region?	Impulsivity and perseverative errors
Which region of the prefrontal cortex is associated with social context and empathy?	Lateral orbitofrontal cortex
A lesion of what cerebral lobe produces incontinence and loss of defecation control?	Frontal lobe (particularly superior frontal gyrus and anterior cingulate)

Which language center is located in the ventrolateral region of the frontal lobe within the dominant hemisphere?	Broca area
A lesion in Broca area produces what symptoms?	Expressive aphasia—loss of motor speech (known as Broca aphasia)
Involvement of adjacent motor cortex can lead to what symptoms?	Apraxia of the face, lips, and tongue, as well as contralateral hemiparesis

TEMPORAL LOBE

What arteries supply the temporal lobe?	Both the middle and posterior cerebral arteries
The primary auditory cortex is located in which fissure?	Sylvian fissure
Where in the temporal lobe is the uncus found?	Inferomedial aspect
A seizure initiated within the uncus produces what type of sensory hallucinations?	Smell and taste
Learning and long-term memory functions are attributed to what medial temporal lobe structures?	Hippocampus and parahippocampal cortex
How many cortical layers are found within the hippocampus and dentate gyrus?	Three layers
What structure(s) connect the left and right temporal lobes?	Corpus callosum and anterior commissure
Meyer loop (or the geniculocalcarine pathway) has visual fibers running through which lobe?	Temporal lobe
A lesion of the amygdala, bilaterally, produces Klüver-Bucy syndrome (in monkeys), which is characterized by what features?	Hypersexuality, hyperphagia, hyperorality, visual agnosia, and fearlessness
Where is Wernicke area located?	Posterior aspect of the superior temporal gyrus
What type of aphasia results from lesions of Wernicke area?	Receptive aphasia

LIMBIC SYSTEM

What are the basic functions associated with the limbic system?	Memory and emotion
What are the structures associated with the basic limbic circuit (Papez circuit)?	Hippocampal formation Mammillary bodies Anterior thalamus (anterior and dorsomedial nuclei) Cingulate gyrus
What other structures are heavily connected to the limbic system?	Amygdala, parahippocampal gyrus, and olfactory bulb
Where are the hippocampus and amygdala located?	Medial temporal lobe
In the Papez circuit, the anterior nuclei of the thalamus receive information from which structure?	Mammillary bodies via the mammillothalamic tract
In the Papez circuit, the anterior thalamic nuclei send efferent projections to what structure?	Cingulate gyrus
What is the name of the white matter tract from the hippocampus to the mammillary bodies?	Fornix

THALAMUS

Which nuclei of the thalamus are considered relay nuclei?	Ventral anterior (VA) Ventral lateral (VL) VPL VPM Lateral geniculate (LGN) Medial geniculate (MGN)
From which brain regions do the VA and VL receive input?	VA: basal ganglia VL: basal ganglia and cerebellum
To what cortical regions do fibers from the VA and VL project?	Motor regions (primary, premotor, and supplementary motor cortex)
What other thalamic nucleus receives input from the basal ganglia?	Centromedian nucleus (CM-IL)

The VPL projects mainly to which cerebral gyrus?	Postcentral gyrus
What type of sensory information is relayed by the LGN?	Vision
The LGN nucleus receives information from what two structures?	1. Retina (via the optic nerve and tract) 2. Primary visual (striate) cortex
In which sensory modality does the MGN play a role?	Hearing
Neurons in the MGN send a large bundle of axons, known as the auditory radiations, to which part of the cerebral cortex?	Transverse temporal (Heschl) gyrus
Which thalamic nucleus sends information to association cortex for sensory integration?	Pulvinar nucleus
What thalamic nucleus has input and output connections with other thalamic nuclei and is involved in the reticular activating system?	Reticular nucleus
What other thalamic nuclei are involved in the reticular activating system?	Intralaminar nuclei

BASAL GANGLIA

What structures make up the striatum?	Caudate nucleus and putamen (dorsal) Nucleus accumbens (ventral striatum)
What structures make up the lentiform nucleus?	Putamen and globus pallidus
What separates the lenticular (lentiform) nuclei from the caudate?	Internal capsule
The basal ganglia is supplied by what arteries?	Lenticulostriate arteries and anterior choroidal artery
What vessel supplies the inner globus pallidus?	Anterior choroidal artery
The claustrum is separated from the lentiform nuclei by what structure?	External capsule
What is the function of the claustrum?	Despite intricate connections with cortical areas, function remains unknown

What is the name of the dopaminergic pathway between the substantia nigra and striatum?	Nigrostriatal pathway

CEREBELLUM

What structure is located at the midline of the cerebellum?	Cerebellar vermis
What is the function of the cerebellar vermis?	Maintaining axial muscle tone and postural control
What neurons send efferent fibers from the cerebellar cortex to the deep nuclei?	Purkinje cells
Which ascending tracts provide "unconscious proprioceptive information" to the cerebellum?	Spinocerebellar and cuneocerebellar tracts
What are some of the symptoms associated with cerebellar lesions?	Ataxia, intention tremor, hypotonia, and loss of coordination
Does a hemispheric lesion of the cerebellum cause contralateral or ipsilateral dysfunction?	Ipsilateral
During development, from what secondary vesicle is the cerebellum derived?	Metencephalon
What are the major functions of the cerebellum?	Coordinate movements, body equilibrium, and muscle tone maintenance
What are some of the symptoms of a lesion in the flocculonodular lobe?	Incoordination and wide-based gait

SPEECH AND LANGUAGE DISORDERS

Which cerebral hemisphere usually contains the major language areas?	Left hemisphere
Where is the planum temporale located?	Superior surface of the temporal lobe posterior to Heschl gyrus
The planum temporale is larger, in most cases, in which cerebral hemisphere?	Left hemisphere

Which language area is located within the planum temporale and superior temporal gyrus?

Wernicke area

Perception of written language is attributed to what cortical region?

Angular gyrus

What is the term used to describe an impairment in the production and/or comprehension of spoken or written language?

Aphasia

Which type of aphasia patient presents with a lack of spoken or written comprehension, an inability to repeat spoken language, but speaks with volumes of words (fluent) devoid of meaning, and is unaware of their deficits?

Wernicke aphasia (receptive)

Where is Wernicke area?

Posterior aspect of the superior temporal gyrus

What are phonemes?

The smallest unit of sound recognized as language

Alexia and agraphia are seen in lesions within what part of the brain?

Inferior parietal lobe

What type of aphasia presents with relatively preserved comprehension, a nonfluent (sparse) use of words, trouble naming objects, possible right-sided weakness, and the patient recognizing their ineptitude?

Broca aphasia (expressive)

What term is used to describe a patient who repeats words or phrases that they hear?

Echolalia

What are neologisms?

Made-up words (or syllables) that are not part of the language

What term describes a defect in articulation despite normal mental functions and intact comprehension of both spoken and written language?

Dysarthria

Patients suffering with agraphia cannot do what?

Communicate through writing

What type of aphasia is produced by destruction of both Broca and Wernicke area as well as a major part of the territory between them?	Global or total aphasia
What is the most common cause of a global aphasia?	Occlusion of the left internal carotid artery or proximal middle cerebral artery
An individual cannot write, repeat, or read and is basically mute. What type of aphasia is present?	Global
What type of visual deficit is sometimes found in patients with global aphasia?	Right homonymous hemianopsia
What type of aphasia occurs by a lesion that separates the receptive and expressive language areas which spares comprehension but leaves the person unable to repeat?	Conduction aphasia
What pathway connecting Wernicke and Broca area is damaged in conduction aphasia?	Arcuate fasciculus
What is the most likely etiology of conduction aphasia?	Occlusion of the posterior temporal branch of the middle cerebral artery
Which aphasia occurs following damage of the cerebral cortex, but preservation of the perisylvian language arc?	Transcortical or isolation aphasias
Describe a transcortical motor aphasia:	Speech is nonfluent, but repetition is intact.
Lesions in what cortical area are associated with transcortical motor aphasia?	Dorsolateral frontal cortex or supplementary motor area
What are the symptoms of transcortical sensory aphasia?	Fluent speech, with poor comprehension, but intact repetition
What lesion causes transcortical sensory aphasia?	Lesions of cortical regions joining temporal, parietal, and occipital lobes
What are some common causes of isolation aphasia?	Anoxia, CO poisoning, and occasionally Alzheimer disease
What condition presents with a full capacity to write fluently, but an inability to read aloud, name colors, or understand written script?	Alexia without agraphia (word blindness)

Where is the site of the typical lesion causing "alexia without agraphia"?

Left geniculocalcarine tract

Patients with alexia without agraphia usually suffer from what visual field defect?

Right homonymous hemianopia

Table 4.2 Features of Common Aphasia

Aphasia	Comprehension	Repetition	Fluency	Associated Symptoms
Wernicke	Poor	Mild	Fluent	Meaningless speech Neologisms
Broca	Preserved	Moderate	Nonfluent	Frustrated speech Hemiparesis
Conduction	Preserved	Poor	Fluent	
Global	Poor	Poor	Nonfluent	All language is affected.

CLINICAL VIGNETTES

Make the diagnosis for the following patients:

A 65-year-old patient with a history of cardiac arrhythmia presents to the ER with right-sided facial paralysis and aphasia. Physical examination reveals dysarthria and nonfluent aphasia. The patient speaks in short phrases lacking words, articles, and conjunctions such as "the, and, if, or but." Comprehension appears to be mostly intact, and the patient shows signs of frustration. ECG demonstrates absent P waves and irregular ventricular rate, suggesting atrial fibrillation. Imaging reveals an ischemic lesion in the left inferior frontal lobe.

Broca aphasia due to thromboembolic occlusion of middle cerebral artery (MCA) branches

A 54-year-old male presents to the ER after an apparent stroke. Physical examination reveals fluent speech, good comprehension, but poor repetition. The patient is unable to repeat the commonly tested phrase "no ifs, ands, or buts." He also appears to have a right superior quadrantanopsia and right-sided limb apraxia. Imaging reveals a lesion involving the white matter between the left superior temporal and inferior frontal cortex.

Conduction aphasia due to ischemia lesion of the arcuate fasciculus

A 64-year-old male with history of HTN, deep venous thrombosis (DVT), and endocarditis suffered a right MCA infarction with a lesion in the parietal lobe diagnosed by MRI 2 years ago. His wife brought him to the office complaining that he has only been eating half of his dinner plate, saying that there is no more food on the plate. He has also stopped shaving the left side of his face. His wife is confused because his vision was not affected by his stroke and previous visual field testing was normal bilaterally. During a line bisection test, you find that he draws the midline on the right side of the line. On line cancellation, he only crosses out lines on the right side.

Left hemineglect due to right parietal lobe lesion

CHAPTER 5

Electrophysiology

RESTING POTENTIAL

What is the approximate resting potential of a neuron?	-70 mV
What is the name for a change in membrane potential toward zero?	Depolarization
What is the name for a change in membrane potential away from zero?	Hyperpolarization
What determines the membrane potential of any cell?	Relative concentration of ions in the cytoplasm and extracellular fluid
What protein maintains the relative concentrations of sodium and potassium?	Na/K-ATPase
What is the name for the potential difference that balances the ionic concentration gradient?	Equilibrium potential (E)
Which two ions have a positive equilibrium potential under physiologic conditions, and would therefore depolarize the cell if made permeable?	1. Sodium 2. Calcium
Which two ions have a negative equilibrium potential under physiologic conditions?	1. Potassium 2. Chloride
Which equation takes into account membrane permeability of multiple ions in order to calculate resting membrane potential?	Goldman equation (derived from Nernst equation)
Resting membrane potential is dominated by permeability to which ion?	Potassium
Which cells are responsible for buffering excess extracellular potassium?	Astrocytes

ACTION POTENTIALS

What is the name of the all-or-none electrical event initiated in the axon hillock, and reliably transmitted over the entire length of the axon?	Action potential
What are the four phases of an action potential?	1. Rising phase 2. Overshoot 3. Falling phase 4. Undershoot (hyperpolarization)
Permeability to which ion is responsible for the rising phase of an action potential?	Sodium
Opening of what type of channels occurs at threshold?	Voltage-gated sodium channels
What event occurs at the peak of an action potential allowing for falling phase to occur?	Inactivation/closing of voltage-gated sodium channels
What important principle of an action potential also depends on inactivation of voltage-gated sodium channels at positive voltages?	Directionality (prevents the action potential from spreading in both directions)
How are action potentials propagated in unmyelinated axons?	Current spreads to depolarize adjacent membranes above threshold.
Are individual action potentials from the same neuron different in terms of shape and peak voltage?	No, they are essentially identical.
Does the peak voltage vary as a function of stimulus strength?	No (stimulus strength increases the frequency)
Permeability of which ion is responsible for the falling phase and undershoot?	Potassium
What is another name for the voltage-gated potassium channels responsible for the falling phase?	Delayed rectifier
What toxin, isolated from the puffer fish, is used to block sodium channels?	Tetrodotoxin
What is the name for the period in which the cell is incapable of firing another action potential, regardless of stimulus?	Absolute refractory period

What is the name of the period following the absolute refractory period in which only a strong stimulus can trigger an action potential? — Relative refractory period

Which refractory period is due to the inactivation of sodium channels? — Absolute refractory period

Which refractory period is due to hyperpolarization? — Relative refractory period

CABLE PROPERTIES

What two properties are most important in determining conduction velocity of an axon?
1. Diameter
2. Myelination

What is the term used to describe resistance to the flow of current down an axon or dendrite? — Internal resistance (axial resistance)

What is the term used to describe resistance to current flow across the membrane? — Membrane resistance

What is the name of the constant defined as the distance over which the membrane voltage falls to 37% of its original value (V_0/e)? — Length constant (space constant)

Which two factors is the length constant dependent on?`
1. Internal resistance
2. Membrane resistance

How does a larger diameter increase conduction velocity? — Decreases internal resistance

What is the term used to describe the storing of charge on either side of the cell membrane? — Membrane capacitance

What is the constant defined as the time it takes for the membrane to charge to 63% of the final voltage? — Time constant

On what two factors is the time constant dependent?
1. Membrane resistance
2. Membrane capacitance

How does myelination increase conduction velocity?	Increases membrane resistance (preventing ion leakage), decreases membrane capacitance
Where is the highest density of voltage-gated sodium channels in a myelinated axon?	Nodes of Ranvier
What is the term used to describe the jumping of action potentials from node to node along myelinated axons?	Saltatory conduction

NEUROTRANSMISSION

How is the strength of a stimulus coded by neurons?	Action potential frequency
What are the three primary anatomic types of synapses?	1. Axodendritic: axon to dendrite 2. Axosomatic: axon to soma (cell body) 3. Axoaxonic: axon to axon
A synapse between dendrites of two neurons would most likely represent what type of synapse?	Electrical synapse
What type of channels, permeable to both ions and small second messengers, are responsible for electrical synapses?	Gap junctions
What are the protein subunits of gap junctions called?	Connexins
Besides nervous tissue, what tissues are especially dependent on gap junctions?	Cardiac and smooth muscles
What is the term for synapses requiring the release of neurotransmitter and binding to postsynaptic receptors for transmitting neural signals?	Chemical synapses
What ion channels are required for release of neurotransmitter when an action potential reaches the presynaptic terminal?	Voltage-gated calcium channels
Which type of neurotransmitters are synthesized in the rough endoplasmic reticulum (rER) and transported to the nerve terminal?	Peptides

Where are neuropeptides found in the synaptic terminal?	Secretory granules
Where are classic amine and amino acid neurotransmitters synthesized?	Cytosol of the synaptic terminal
Where are amine and amino acid neurotransmitters found in the presynaptic terminal?	Synaptic vesicles
What mitochondrial enzyme is capable of metabolizing biogenic amine neurotransmitters?	Monoamine oxidase (MAO)
What postsynaptic protein performs a similar function?	Catechol-O-methyltransferase (COMT)
What is the cellular process responsible for release of neurotransmitter?	Exocytosis
Recycling of membrane involves fusion of endocytic vesicles with which organelle?	Endosome
Which proteins, expressed on vesicles, regulate the organelles with which a vesicle is destined to fuse?	COP-I and II
What proteins are responsible for the fusion of vesicle and cell membranes?	SNAREs (v-SNARE for vesicle and t-SNARE for target)
Which injectable cosmetic agent inhibits fusion of SNARE proteins?	Botulinum toxin
What are the actual sites of neurotransmitter release called?	Active zones

NEUROTRANSMITTERS

Of the classic neurotransmitters, which are amino acids?	Glutamate, glycine, and gamma-amino butyric acid (GABA)
What is the primary excitatory neurotransmitter in the central nervous system (CNS)?	Glutamate
Which neurotransmitters are classified as the biogenic amines?	Acetylcholine (ACh), dopamine (DA), norepinephrine (NE), epinephrine (Epi), serotonin (5-HT), and histamine

Which of the biogenic amines are classified as catecholamines?	Dopamine, norepinephrine, and epinephrine
From what amino acid can all of the catecholamines be synthesized?	Tyrosine
What are the critical enzymes in the synthesis of each of the catecholamines?	Dopamine: tyrosine hydroxylase (TH) Norepinephrine: dopamine-β-hydroxylase (DBH) Epinephrine: phentolamine-*N*-methyltransferase (PNMT)
Which pigment is also associated with catecholamine metabolism?	Melanin
What is the amino acid precursor of serotonin?	Tryptophan
What molecule found in the pineal gland is also associated with tryptophan metabolism?	Melatonin
What critical component for oxidative phosphorylation is associated with the tryptophan metabolic pathways?	Niacin
From which amine acid is histamine derived?	Histidine
What is the word for the fixed amount of neurotransmitter released from an individual vesicle?	Quantum
What is the phrase describing the postsynaptic response to a quantum of neurotransmitter?	Miniature postsynaptic potential
Where is the major norepinephrine nucleus sending out diffuse projections throughout the CNS?	Locus coeruleus
What color is locus coeruleus as a result of melanin as a byproduct of catecholamine metabolism?	Blue
What are the major serotonergic nuclei of the brainstem?	Raphe nuclei
What are the major dopaminergic nuclei?	Ventral tegmental area (VTA) and substantia nigra (SN)

Dopaminergic transmission from the VTA to the nucleus accumbens is implicated in what type of clinical problem?	Addiction
Which diseases are associated with disturbances of dopaminergic transmission?	Parkinson disease, schizophrenia, and attention-deficit hyperactivity disorder (ADHD)
What are the major acetylcholinergic nuclei?	Nucleus basalis of Meynert and medial septal nuclei
Loss of neurons in the major acetylcholinergic nuclei is associated with what dementing illness?	Alzheimer disease

RECEPTORS

What are the two basic types of neurotransmitter receptors?	1. Ionotropic 2. Metabotropic
Which type of receptor acts through the opening of ion channels?	Ionotropic
Which type of receptor acts through G-proteins, second messengers, and signaling pathways?	Metabotropic
Which type of receptor has a faster response?	Ionotropic
Which type of receptor has a longer lasting response?	Metabotropic
A receptor that is coupled to the phosphorylation of a potassium channel, making it more likely to open, would fall into which category of receptor?	Metabotropic
What is the term used to describe receptors on the presynaptic terminal which provide regulatory feedback on the amount of neurotransmitter being released?	Autoreceptors
Classify both the nicotinic and muscarinic ACh receptors as either ionotropic or metabotropic:	Nicotinic: ionotropic Muscarinic: metabotropic

What disease characterized by muscle weakness and double vision is sometimes caused by tumors or hyperplasia of the thymus?	Myasthenia gravis
What is the mechanism behind the weakness associated with myasthenia gravis?	Autoantibodies to the ACh receptor
What radiologic finding is associated with myasthenia gravis?	Enlarged thymus due to lymphoid hyperplasia
What is the name of the diagnostic test for myasthenia gravis using edrophonium?	Tensilon test
What class of drugs is used in the treatment of myasthenia gravis?	Acetylcholinesterase inhibitors
What is the function of acetylcholinesterase?	Breakdown ACh in the synaptic cleft
Acetylcholinesterase inhibitors are also used in the treatment of which common dementia associated with disruption of ACh transmission?	Alzheimer disease
What paraneoplastic syndrome in small cell lung cancer is clinically similar to myasthenia gravis?	Lambert-Eaton syndrome
Autoantibodies against which protein are made in Lambert-Eaton syndrome?	Calcium channels—preventing ACh release
What additional dysfunction occurs in Lambert-Eaton syndrome as a result of deficient ACh release?	Parasympathetic dysfunction
What is different about the presentation of Lambert-Eaton syndrome compared to myasthenia gravis?	Lambert-Eaton syndrome rarely involves oculomotor weakness at onset, and causes greater weakness in legs than arms.
What are the downstream effects of each of the G-proteins associated with metabotropic receptors?	G_s: activates adenylyl cyclase $\rightarrow$ increases cAMP G_i: inhibits adenylyl cyclase $\rightarrow$ decreases cAMP G_q: activates PLC $\rightarrow$ increases IP_3 (inositol-1,4,5 triphosphate), DAG dracylglycerol), and intracellular calcium

What word is used to describe an ionotropic receptor that brings the cell closer to threshold voltage on binding of neurotransmitter?	Excitatory
In general, channels selective for which ions are opened by binding of ligand to excitatory ionotropic receptors?	Sodium and potassium, but sodium current overpowers potassium
What is the term used to describe the change in voltage associated with the activation of excitatory receptors?	Excitatory postsynaptic potential (EPSP)
What is the term used to describe the change in voltage during activation of inhibitory receptors?	Inhibitory postsynaptic potential (IPSP)
Postsynaptic potentials have to travel along which type of neurites?	Dendrites
Integration of synaptic inputs occurs at which part of the neuron?	Axon hillock/initial segment
What are the two types of integration that occur at the axon hillock?	1. Spatial summation 2. Temporal summation
Which type of summation involves summing simultaneous postsynaptic potentials from multiple dendrites?	Spatial summation
Which type of summation involves summing of a rapid series of postsynaptic potentials from an individual dendrite?	Temporal summation
Channels selective for which ions are opened by activation of inhibitory ionotropic receptors?	Chloride
Which receptors are ionotropic, inhibitory, and chloride channels?	$GABA_A$ receptors in the brain, and glycine receptors in the spinal cord
How are $GABA_A$ receptors excitatory in the developing brain?	Different ion concentrations causing chloride-mediated depolarization
What two classes of drugs activate the $GABA_A$ receptor?	1. Benzodiazepines 2. Barbiturates
What other intoxicating substance is believed to enhance GABA conductance?	Ethanol

What are the different types of ionotropic glutamate receptors?	AMPA/kainate and NMDA (*N*-methyl-D-aspartic acid) receptors
Which type of glutamate receptors is responsible for long-term potentiation (LTP)?	NMDA receptors
What cognitive process is often attributed to LTP?	Long-term memory formation
In which axonal pathway is LTP classically studied as a molecular mechanism of memory?	Schaffer collateral pathway between CA3 and CA1 of the hippocampus
Who was the patient made famous by an inability to form new memories (anterograde amnesia) after removal of both hippocampi?	Henry Molaison (H.M.)
What two factors make NMDA receptors unique?	1. Require both ligand-binding and depolarization 2. Allow calcium influx
What divalent ion is responsible for voltage gating of the NMDA receptor?	Magnesium
Which receptors are responsible for generating the depolarization required for NMDA activation?	AMPA/kainate receptors
What retrograde messenger is believed to be involved in LTP?	Nitric oxide
What are the downstream pathways involved in regulating changes in protein expression required for LTP?	CAMKII → PKA → cAMP → CREB
What two properties make LTP a likely molecular mechanism for memory?	1. Associativity: weak stimuli can be strengthened if associated with strong stimuli. 2. Cooperativity: requirement of a suprathreshold stimulus.
What process, also requiring calcium and protein synthesis, is responsible for weakening certain synapses?	Long-term depression (LTD)

CLINICAL VIGNETTES

Make the diagnosis for the following patients:

A 24-year-old woman comes to your office complaining of progressive weakness, especially in the facial and neck muscles. She sometimes has double vision while reading and occasionally feels a general weakness. On physical examination, she has a symmetric reduction in proximal muscle strength, particularly with repeated movements, and ptosis of the eyelids. Cranial nerve testing reveals facial muscle weakness and nystagmus. Tensilon test is positive, as is antiacetylcholine receptor antibody titre. Computed tomography (CT) demonstrates an enlarged thymus.

Myasthenia gravis

A 54-year-old male smoker with a 60-pack-year history (2 packs per day × 30 years) complains of progressive weakness in the muscles of his hips and thighs. On physical examination, the patient has proximal limb weakness and reduced reflexes. Tensilon and antiacetylcholine antibody tests are negative. Chest CT reveals findings suggestive of lung cancer. Sputum cytology demonstrates small round cells with dark nucleus and little cytoplasm.

Lambert-Eaton syndrome secondary to small cell lung cancer

CHAPTER 6

Sensory Systems

SOMATOSENSORY SYSTEM

Table 6.1 Somatosensory Receptors

Receptor	Fiber Group	Modality
Meissner	$A\alpha/\beta$	Stroking
Merkel	$A\alpha/\beta$	Pressure
Pacinian	$A\alpha/\beta$	Vibration
Ruffini	$A\alpha/\beta$	Stretch
Cold nociceptors	C	Cold
Heat nociceptors	$A\delta$	Hot
Fast pain (sharp)	$A\delta$	Sharp pain
Slow pain (burning)	C	Slow pain
Muscle spindle	Ia, II	Muscle stretch
Golgi tendon organ (GTO)	Ib	Muscle tension

Name the epidermal receptor described below:

> Onion-like receptor responsive to vibration — Pacinian corpuscle

> Primary receptor responsible for two-point discrimination — Meissner corpuscle

> Slowly adapting receptor responsible for pressure sensation — Ruffini ending

Which epidermal receptors adapt rapidly? — Meissner corpuscle and pacinian corpuscle

Which epidermal receptors adapt slowly to constant stimulation? — Merkel disks and Ruffini ending

Which pain fibers are myelinated, $A\delta$ or C fibers? — $A\delta$: responsible for "first pain"

Table 6.2 Somatosensory Tracts

System	Function	Receptors	Course
Anterolateral (ALS)	Pain and temperature Crude touch	Free nerve endings	1. Dorsal root ganglion 2. Tract of Lissauer 3. Dorsal horn laminae I and II 4. Ventral white commissure (decussation) 5. Spinothalamic tract 6. Ventral posterolateral nucleus (VPL) 7. Postcentral gyrus
Dorsal column–medial lemniscal (DC/ML)	Vibration Pressure Discriminative touch Conscious proprioception	Pacinian Meissner Merkel disks Ruffini ending Spindle and GTO	1. Dorsal root ganglion 2. Dorsal columns 3. Cuneate and gracile nuclei 4. Internal arcuate fibers (decussation) 5. Medial lemniscus 6. VPL 7. Postcentral gyrus
Dorsal spinocerebellar tract (DSCT)	Unconscious proprioception (C8 and below)	Joint receptors Spindles GTO	1. Dorsal root ganglion 2. Clarke column (C8–L3) 3. DSCT 4. Inferior cerebellar peduncle 5. Cerebellum (Ipsilateral)

Cuneocerebellar tract (CCT)	Unconscious proprioception (C7 and above)	Joint receptors Spindles GTO	1. Dorsal root ganglion 2. Accessory cuneate nucleus 3. CCT 4. Inferior cerebellar peduncle 5. Cerebellum (Ipsilateral)
Trigeminal (face)	Pain and temperature	Free nerve endings	1. Trigeminal ganglion 2. Spinal trigeminal tract 3. Spinal trigeminal nucleus 4. Trigeminothalamic tract (majority decussate) 5. Ventral posteromedial nucleus (VPM) 6. Postcentral gyrus
	Vibration Pressure Discriminative touch	Pacinian Meissner Merkel disks Ruffini endings	1. Trigeminal ganglion 2. Principle sensory nucleus of CN V 3. Trigeminothalamic tract (ventral decussates) 4. VPM 5. Postcentral gyrus
	Proprioception	Spindle and GTO	1. Mesencephalic nucleus of CN V 2. Trigeminothalamic tract 3. VPM 4. Postcentral gyrus

*First-order neurons of the proprioceptive division of CN V are located in the mesencephalic nucleus of CN V. Jaw jerk reflex is mediated by direct monosynaptic reflex with the motor nucleus of CN V.

VISUAL SYSTEM

Which photoreceptors carry black and white information?	Rods
What is another name for "night vision"?	Scotopic vision
Which photoreceptors carry color information?	Cones
What is another name for "daytime vision"?	Photopic vision
In what region of the retina are cones concentrated?	Fovea
Which type of photoreceptors become easily saturated, but can detect a single photon?	Rods

Table 6.3 Rods vs Cones

Photoreceptor	Rod	Cone
Sensitivity	High	Low
Temporal resolution	Low (slow response)	High (fast response)
Acuity	Low	High
Color	Achromatic	Chromatic: three types

What do you call the tonic activation of Na current through cyclic guanosine monophosphate (cGMP)-gated channels in the dark?	Dark current
What is the net effect of dark current?	Tonic depolarization
What is the effect of light on dark current?	Phasic hyperpolarization
What molecule activated by light changes 11-cis retinal to all trans retinal?	Rhodopsin
Which cranial nerve carries visual information?	CN II: optic nerve
Which cells make up the optic nerve?	Axons of retinal ganglion cells
Which cells are the first in the visual pathway capable of firing action potentials?	Ganglion cells

Through which skull opening does the optic nerve pass?	Optic canal
What physical examination finding is found in patients with optic nerve damage?	Marcus-Gunn pupil (swinging flashlight test)
A Marcus Gunn pupil is indicative of damage to which limb of the pupillary reflex?	The afferent limb (optic nerve)
What cells myelinate the axons of the ganglion cells?	Oligodendrocytes
To which division of the central nervous system (CNS) does the optic nerve belong?	Diencephalon
What are the ten layers of the retina from outside inward?	1. Pigment epithelium 2. Layer of rods and cones 3. Outer limiting membrane 4. Outer nuclear 5. Outer plexiform 6. Inner nuclear 7. Inner plexiform 8. Ganglion cell layer 9. Layer of optic nerve fibers 10. Inner limiting membrane

Which cells reside in the following layers of the retina:

Outer nuclear	Photoreceptors
Outer plexiform	Horizontal cells
Inner nuclear	Bipolar cells
Inner plexiform	Amacrine cells
Between which layers does retinal detachment most often occur?	Pigment epithelium and layer of rods and cones
What is the signaling order of the vertical pathway in the retina?	Photoreceptors → bipolar cells → ganglion cells
What type of receptive field is created by the lateral inhibition provided by horizontal and amacrine cells?	Center-surround
Which cells in the vertical pathway have center-surround receptive fields?	Bipolar and ganglion cells
What is the purpose of the center-surround configuration of the retina?	Contrast and edge detection

What is the primary blood supply of the retina?

Central retinal artery

What phrase is used to describe sudden, transient visual loss?

Amaurosis fugax

What is the most common cause of this transient blindness?

Atherosclerotic stenosis of the internal carotid circulation

What is the funduscopic examination finding of amaurosis fugax?

Hollenhorst plaque (cholesterol embolus)

What parts of the retina receive light from the left visual hemifield?

Left nasal and right temporal hemiretina (see Fig. 6.1 for more details)

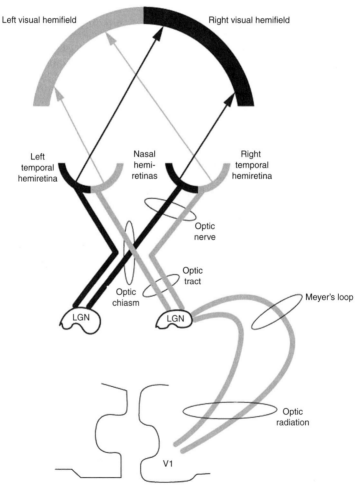

Figure 6.1   Schematic diagram of information flow within the visual system.

How do you test the integrity of a patient's retina?

Confrontational visual field testing

What are the two most common types of retinal ganglion cells?

1. M cells (for magni, also known as parasol cells)
2. P cells (for parvi, also known as midget cells)

Table 6.4 Magnocellular vs Parvocellular Ganglion Cells

	M cells	P cells
Receptive field	Large	Small
Contrast sensitivity	High	Low
Adaptation	Rapid	Slow
Spatial resolution	Low	High
Color	No	Yes
Function	Edges and movement	Fine detail

Information from which part of the visual fields crosses in the optic chiasm?

Temporal/peripheral

Crossing in the optic chiasm allows for all information from one side of visual space to enter which side of the optic tract?

Contralateral side

Which thalamic nucleus receives visual information from retinal ganglion cells?

Lateral geniculate nucleus (LGN)

Which layers of the LGN receive uncrossed information from the ipsilateral eye?

Layers 2, 3, and 5

Which layers of the LGN receive crossed information from the contralateral eye?

Layers 1, 4, and 6

Which layers of the LGN receive magnocellular information (from M cells)?

Layers 1 and 2

Which layers of the LGN receive parvocellular information (from P cells)?

Layers 3 through 6

List the visual pathway from retina to cortex:	• Ganglion cells of the retina • Optic nerve • Optic chiasm • Optic tract • LGN • Optic radiation (geniculocarcarine tract) • Visual cortex (striate cortex)
What are the two portions of the optic radiation?	1. Temporal lobe portion (Meyer loop) 2. Parietal lobe portion
What pathway is used for color and object recognition?	Parvocellular (see Table 6.5 for more information)
List the steps in the parvocellular (what) pathway:	See Table 6.5 for answers
List the steps in the magnocellular (where) pathway:	See Table 6.5 for answers

Table 6.5 Central Visual Pathway

Pathway	Parvocellular	Magnocellular
Ganglion cell	P cell (midget)	M cell (parasol)
LGN layer	Layers 3 through 6	Layers 1 and 2
V1 layer	Layer 4Cβ	4Cα
Projection from layer 4C	Layers 2 and 3	Layer 4b
V2 region	Thin stripe and interstripe	Thick stripe
Processing stream	Ventral stream	Dorsal stream
What or where?	What (color and object)	Where (motion and contrast)

Lesion to which cortical region causes inability to recognize objects, known as agnosia?	IT (inferotemporal cortex)
What is the specific inability to recognize faces seen in a subset of IT lesions called?	Prosopagnosia

A lesion to what region of cortex causes an inability to perceive motion, known as motor blindness?   V5

A lesion in what region of cortex causes a lack of color vision, known as achromatopsia?   V4

Achromatopsia can also be due to a congenital lack of which type of photoreceptor?   Cones

What visual deficits are caused by lesions to the following:

Optic nerve	Ipsilateral blindness
Left optic tract	Right homonymous hemianopia
Lateral optic chiasm (bilaterally)	Binasal hemianopia
Medial optic chiasm	Bitemporal hemianopia
Left Meyer loop (also called left temporal optic radiation)	Right upper quadrantanopia
Left parietal radiation	Right lower quadrantopia
Left visual cortex (area 17)	Right homonymous hemianopia (macular sparing depending on lesion)

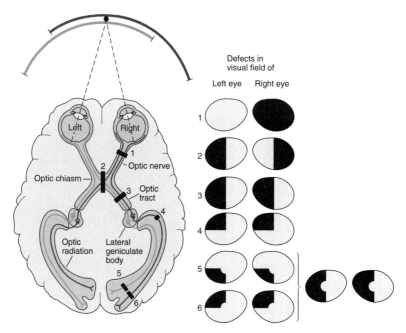

Figure 6.2   Deficits in the visual field produced by lesions at various points in the visual pathway. (Reproduced with permission from Kandel ER, Schwartz JH, Jessell ST, eds. *Principles of Neural Science.* 4th ed. New York, NY: McGraw-Hill; 2000: 544.)

What pathology is suspected in a patient with binasal hemianopia?	Calcification of the internal carotid arteries
What pathology is suspected in a patient with bitemporal hemianopia?	Pituitary adenomas and craniopharyngiomas
What syndrome is suspected in a patient with bilateral cortical damage who is blind but denies blindness and confabulates?	Anton syndrome
A lesion to what region of cortex causes sensory hemineglect, in which a patient ignores one side of space, despite normal visual fields?	Nondominant parietal lobe
What disease process may spare central vision and destroy all peripheral fields?	End-stage glaucoma
Occlusion of which major vessel leads to cortical blindness with macular sparing?	Posterior cerebral artery (PCA)
Collateral supply from which vessel is believed to allow macular sparing in PCA occlusion?	Middle cerebral artery (MCA)
Loss of central vision with peripheral sparing, known as central scotoma, is seen in what feature of multiple sclerosis?	Retrobulbar optic neuritis

AUDITORY SYSTEM

What frequencies do humans hear?	20 to 20,000 Hz
What is the name of the inner ear structure responsible for hearing?	Cochlea
What bones are responsible for transmitting sound from the tympanic membrane to the cochlea?	Malleus, incus, and stapes
What part of the cochlea does the stapes directly contact?	Oval window
What is the site of sound transduction from mechanical to electrical input?	Organ of Corti

What part of the cochlea detects high frequency?	Proximal basilar membrane, known as the base
What is the term used to describe the organization of auditory information by sound frequency?	Tonotopic organization
Which type of hair cells are the primary processors of sound?	Inner hair cells
Which type of hair cells are the primary amplification system?	Outer hair cells
Information from which type of hair cell travels along myelinated axons of bipolar cells, terminating at the cochlear nuclei?	Inner hair cells
Which ion is responsible for depolarization in the inner ear?	Potassium
How is this possible?	The concentration gradient favors potassium influx from the endolymph.
How are the channels that allow potassium influx opened as a result of sound?	Displacement of stereocilia causes mechanical deformation of ion channels located at tip links between stereocilia.
List the structures in the auditory neural pathway from inner ear to primary auditory cortex.	1. Hair cells in organ of Corti 2. Bipolar cells of spiral ganglion 3. Cochlear nerve (CN VIII) 4. Cochlear nuclei 5. Trapezoid body 6. Superior olivary complex 7. Lateral lemniscus 8. Inferior colliculus 9. Medial geniculate body 10. Auditory radiation 11. Primary auditory cortex
What is the name of the decussating tract from the cochlear nuclei to the contralateral superior olivary nuclei?	Trapezoid body
What cluster of nuclei in the caudal pons is the first to receive binaural input, and is responsible for horizontal localization of sound?	Superior olivary complex

What characteristics of binaural auditory input are compared in sound localization?	Differences in interaural timing and sound intensity
What are other names for the primary auditory cortex?	Transverse temporal gyri of Heschl or Brodmann areas 41 and 42
What are the two types of deafness?	1. Conduction deafness 2. Sensorineural
Which type of deafness is defined as difficulty getting the sound waves from the air through to the inner ear?	Conductive
Which type of deafness is defined as difficulty getting the sound signal from the inner ear to the brain?	Sensorineural
What is the most common cause of conduction deafness in children?	Otitis media
What is the cause of otitis media?	Dysfunctional eustachian tubes— normally drain the middle ear into the nasopharynx
How does otitis media cause conduction deafness?	Excess middle ear fluid
What is the most common cause of sensorineural hearing loss in the elderly?	Presbycusis
Which frequencies become difficult to hear as a result of presbycusis?	High frequency
Which parts of speech become difficult to hear as a result of presbycusis?	Consonants
Which tuning fork is used for Weber and Rinne hearing tests?	512 Hz
Which fork is used to test vibratory sensation?	128 Hz
Which test involves placing the tuning fork at middle of the forehead and asking where they hear the sound?	Weber
Which test involves placing the tuning fork behind the ear and testing air versus bone conduction?	Rinne

Which test is more useful for detecting gross hearing loss?	Weber
Which test is used to categorize hearing loss?	Rinne

What is the significance of the following hearing test findings:

Sound heard equally in both ears on Weber test	Normal (see Table 6.6 for more information)
Sound heard louder in one ear on Weber test	Ipsilateral conductive or contralateral sensorineural loss
Air conduction better than bone on Rinne	Normal or ipsilateral sensorineural loss
Bone conduction better than air on Rinne	Ipsilateral conductive loss

Table 6.6 Webber vs Rinne Test

	Weber	Rinne
Normal	Heard equally well	Air louder than bone
Conductive	Lateralizes* to bad ear	Bone louder than air
Sensorineural	Lateralizes* to good ear	Air louder than bone

*Lateralizes to = is louder on that side.

What form of conductive hearing loss is caused by immobile middle ear bones?	Otosclerosis
How do you test hearing in an infant?	Brain stem auditory evoked potentials
What conditions in adults can cause abnormal auditory evoked potentials?	Multiple sclerosis or acoustic neuromas

TASTE

What are the four primary tastes?	1. Salty 2. Sour 3. Sweet 4. Bitter
Which tastes primarily use ions for signal transduction?	Salty and sour
Which tastes primarily use G-proteins for signal transduction?	Sweet and bitter
What ion is the signal for salty foods?	Na^+: Na ions enter via a membrane channel and depolarize the receptor.
What ion is the signal for sour foods?	H^+: H ions also enter via a membrane channel to depolarize the receptor.
How do sweet foods activate signal transduction?	Second messengers, including G_{gust}
What do we call the taste of monosodium glutamate (MSG)?	Umami
What do you call a lack of taste?	Ageusia
List the common causes of ageusia:	• Smoking • Peripheral CN VII lesion • Chorda tympani lesion in the middle ear • CN IX lesion
Which nerve carries taste information from the following structures:	
Anterior two-thirds of tongue	Chorda tympani (CN VII)
Posterior one-third of tongue	CN IX
Epiglottis	CN X
Which nucleus of the thalamus receives taste information?	VPM
In which cortical regions is the primary gustatory cortex found?	Insula and operculum

OLFACTION

Which G-protein do odorants, or smells, activate for signal transduction?	G_{olf} ("olf" for olfactory)
Onto what specific cells do olfactory receptors synapse in the glomeruli of the olfactory bulb?	Mitral and tufted cells
Which interneurons in the olfactory bulb help support the glomeruli?	Periglomerular cells and granule cells
With which other neural system is the olfactory system tightly coupled?	Limbic system
What is the olfactory pathway's unique relationship with the thalamus?	Synapses in cortical areas before the thalamus—no thalamic relay
What epithelial cells give olfactory nerves their unique ability to proliferate following injury?	Basal cells
What other neurons have been shown to proliferate after damage?	Granule cells of the hippocampus
What word is defined as a lack of smell?	Anosmia
Trauma to what part of the skull can cause anosmia?	The cribriform plate
How does bilateral anosmia usually present in a patient?	Loss of taste
What disease is caused by large lesions, most often meningiomas, of the olfactory sulcus region?	Foster-Kennedy syndrome
What are the signs of Foster-Kennedy syndrome?	Anosmia, ipsilateral optic atrophy, and contralateral papilledema
What disease is marked by an absence of olfactory bulbs due to insufficient migration of gonadotropin-releasing hormone (GnRH) neurons and results in hypogonadotropic hypogonadism?	Kallmann syndrome

VESTIBULAR SYSTEM

What are the two parts of the vestibular labyrinth?	1. Semicircular canals 2. Otolith organs
What part of the labyrinth detects linear acceleration, including gravity?	Otolith organs: utricle and saccule
Otolith organs are programmed to detect the movement of what substance?	Otoliths (or otoconia): calcium carbonate stones
What part of the labyrinth detects angular acceleration?	Semicircular canals: lateral, anterior, and posterior
What substance fills the membranous organs of the labyrinth?	Endolymph
What substance surrounds the membranous organs of the labyrinth?	Perilymph
While the dominant ion in perilymph is sodium, what is the dominant ion in endolymph?	Potassium
What type of cells embedded in the cupula of the crista ampullaris detects movement of the endolymph?	Hair cells
What are the two types of structures that make up the hair cells?	1. One long kinocilium 2. Several shorter stereocilia
Flow of endolymph that pushes stereocilia away from the kinocilium produces what response?	Inhibition of firing
Flow of endolymph that pushes stereocilia toward the kinocilium produces what response?	Excitation and release of neurotransmitter
Movement of endolymph toward the ampulla in each canal causes what response?	Excitation
Quick rotation of the head to the right causes what response in the hair cells of the right labyrinth?	Excitation
Activation of hair cells leads to activation of the vestibular nuclei by what cells?	Bipolar cells that comprise Scarpa ganglion

Where is information from the vestibular nuclei sent?	Spinal cord, cerebellum, extraocular motor nuclei, thalamus, and other vestibular nuclei
What uncrossed descending tract originating at the lateral vestibular nucleus restores and maintains posture by stimulating motor neurons of the proximal limb musculature?	Lateral vestibulospinal tract
What bilateral projection from the medial vestibular nucleus maintains head position by innervating the motor neurons of the neck muscles?	Medial vestibulospinal tract
What is another name for this tract?	Descending medial longitudinal fasciculus
What region of the cerebellum receives vestibular input?	Flocculonodular lobe and vermis
Visual information from what structure is integrated with vestibular input in order to maintain balance and eye movements?	Superior colliculus
What reflex, mediated by the vestibular system, stabilizes visual images relative to changing head position?	Vestibulo-ocular reflex
How is the vestibulo-ocular reflex tested clinically in comatose patients?	Caloric testing
What is the term used to describe slow horizontal movement of the eyes followed by a quick snapping back?	Nystagmus
What are the three types of nystagmus?	1. Postrotatory 2. Optokinetic 3. Caloric
What is the mnemonic used to remember normal caloric responses in a comatose patient?	COWS (Cold Opposite/Warm Same) referring to the fast phase of nystagmus. The patient looks toward the ear when irrigated with cold water, but away from an ear with warm water. The fast phase of nystagmus is in the opposite direction.

What happens when cold water is irrigated into the right ear of a patient with a lesion in the right pons affecting the abducens nucleus?

Patient does not look toward the irrigated ear.

What happens when cold water is irrigated into the left ear of a patient with a lesion of the right medial longitudinal fasciculus?

The left eye abducts, but the right eye fails to adduct.

Eye movements while looking out the window of a moving car or train fall under which category of nystagmus?

Optokinetic

What causes postrotatory nystagmus?

Inertia of the fluid in the semicircular canals

What is the oculocephalic reflex?

Also known as the doll's eye maneuver, an unconscious patient's head is rotated and vestibular input keeps the eyes fixed on the same target.

Describe how vestibular stimulation causes conjugate lateral gaze:

The vestibular nuclei stimulate the ipsilateral oculomotor nucleus and contralateral abducens nucleus. Oculomotor stimulation drives the adduction by the ipsilateral medial rectus, while the abducens nucleus drives abduction of the contralateral eye by the lateral rectus.

If you turn the head to the right, which vestibular nuclei are stimulated, and which direction will the gaze shift?

Right vestibular nucleus is stimulated causing the eyes to look left.

VERTIGO

What is vertigo?

The sensation that either you or the room is spinning

What is the most common cause of vertigo in adults?

Benign paroxysmal positional vertigo (BPPV)

What condition causes vertigo that is brought on by sudden position changes (rolling over in bed) that usually lasts less than a minute?

BPPV

What is the underlying cause of vertigo in classic BPPV?	Canalolithiasis
What is the standard clinical test for BPPV that may elicit rotatory nystagmus?	Dix-Hallpike test
How is the test performed?	In seated position, rotate head 45°, lay the patient down with head slightly extended, and observe eye movements.
What condition causes vertigo due to inflammation of the canals secondary to drugs or infection?	Labyrinthitis
What condition causes episodic vertigo, tinnitus, hearing loss, and sensation of ear fullness?	Ménière disease
What tumor causes vertigo, tinnitus, and hearing loss?	Acoustic neuroma (schwannoma)

CLINICAL VIGNETTES

Make the diagnosis for the following patients:

A 65-year-old male with history of type 2 diabetes (NIDDM), coronary artery disease (CAD), obesity, HTN, and hyperlipidemia presents with sudden onset of unilateral blindness that lasted 10 minutes before returning to normal. The patient described a "curtain" coming down over his left eye while he was driving the previous day. Physical examination revealed blood pressure of 165/95, and the remainder of examination was normal other than slight carotid bruit heard over left internal carotid artery. On funduscopic exam, there was a bright yellow plaque found at the bifurcation of an arteriole.

Amaurosis fugax with Hollenhorst plaque

A 1-year-old female with history of recurrent otitis media presents with increased irritability and fever. Her parents state that she has not been responding when they call her name. A Weber test is found to lateralize to the right ear. A Rinne test reveals air over bone conduction on the left and bone over air conduction on the right side. On otoscopic examination, you find bulging erythematous tympanic membranes (TM).

Otitis media with conductive hearing loss on the right

A 72-year-old male, retired factory worker with no significant PMH is brought to the office by his wife. She complains of increasing hearing loss in her husband, but he insists that she always mumbles. She claims that he has progressively lost the ability to understand what people are saying in conversation, particularly in noisy settings. All routine laboratory tests are WNL. A Weber test reveals no laterality. A Rinne test reveals air over bone bilaterally. Audiometry demonstrates a bilateral loss of hearing in the high frequency range. Imaging studies are unremarkable.

Presbycusis

A 35-year-old boxer complains of problems with his tongue. He was knocked out by his opponent in a fight 1 week ago. He complains that food seems to taste bland. On physical examination, testing of sweet, salty, sour, and bitter tastes reveals no specific taste or sensory loss in the tongue. However, he was unable to smell any of the odors presented in either nostril. On inquiry, the patient later recalls having a runny nose the day after his fight, but does not recall any other symptoms of a common cold. He described the fluid as clear and thin. X-ray images confirmed the suspected diagnosis.

Anosmia secondary to fracture of the cribriform plate

CHAPTER 7

Motor Systems

Table 7.1 Motor Deficit Terminology

Terminology	Motor Deficit
Paralysis	Complete loss of voluntary movement
-plegia	Complete loss of voluntary movement
-paresis	Partial loss of voluntary movement
Paraplegia	Complete loss of lower limb voluntary movement
Hemiparesis	Partial loss of voluntary movement on one side of the body

Table 7.2 Scoring of Muscle Strength

Normal strength	5
Movement against gravity plus resistance	4
Movement against gravity only	3
Unable to resist gravity	2
Muscle contraction without movement	1
No sign of contraction	0

Table 7.3 Scoring of Reflexes

Absent response	0
Trace response	1
Normal response	2
Brisk response	3
Nonsustained clonus	4
Sustained clonus	5

What is another sign of hyperreflexia?	Spreading to other muscle groups

SPINAL CONTROL

What are the components of a motor unit?	Lower motor neuron Motor neuron axon Muscle fibers innervated
How is the power of a movement increased?	Recruitment of additional motor units
What are the other names for an α-motorneuron?	Lower motor neuron Anterior horn cell
What genetic disease involves the selective loss of anterior horn neurons?	Spinal muscular atrophy (SMA)
What is another name for the most severe form of SMA?	Werdnig-Hoffman disease
What protein is deficient in SMA?	Survival of motor neuron (SMN)—a nucleolar protein
Which muscle fibers are innervated by α-motorneurons?	Extrafusal fibers
Which motor neurons innervate intrafusal fibers?	γ-Motorneurons
What sensory afferents regulate the activity of γ-motorneurons?	Ia afferents from muscles spindles
What are the two components of the muscle spindle apparatus?	1. Nuclear bag 2. Nuclear chain
Describe the order of synapses involved in a myotactic (monosynaptic) reflex:	Ia afferent from muscle spindle innervates α-motorneuron α-Motorneuron innervates muscle
What is the term used to describe the inhibitory innervation of antagonist muscles?	Reciprocal inhibition
What neurotransmitter mediates inhibition of antagonist muscles by spinal interneurons?	Glycine

What type of inhibition is mediated by motor neurons exciting inhibitory interneurons as a negative feedback mechanism?	Recurrent inhibition
What type of spinal neuron is responsible for providing recurrent inhibition?	Renshaw cells
What sensory apparatus is used to regulate tension of muscle fibers during contraction?	Golgi tendon organ (GTO)
Where are GTOs found?	Encapsulated in the connective tissue of tendons
What kind of innervation do GTOs provide to the primary muscle contracting?	Inhibitory innervation via disynaptic reflex
What protective function do GTOs serve?	Prevent excess muscle tension that would cause tearing
Describe how different regions of the ventral horn control various muscle groups:	Medial: axial muscles Lateral: limb muscles Dorsal: flexors Ventral: extensors
What is the term used to describe involuntary muscle twitching?	Fasciculations
What are the key features of lower motor neuron disease?	Flaccidity Hypotonia Atrophy Areflexia Fasciculations
What are common causes of lower motor neuron disease?	Traumatic severing of motor axons Poliomyelitis

CORTICAL CONTROL

What is the major descending motor pathway from the cerebral cortex?	Corticospinal tract
What is another commonly used name for the corticospinal tract?	Pyramidal tract

From which cortical areas do the corticospinal tracts originate?	Primary motor cortex: area 4 Premotor area: area 6 Primary somatosensory cortex: areas 3, 1, and 2
What is the function of the premotor area?	Planning of complex motor tasks
Into which two regions is the premotor area divided?	1. Supplementary motor cortex 2. Premotor cortex
What are the functions of these motor regions?	Supplementary: planning of willed movements Premotor: planning of sensory-guided movements
What thalamic nucleus is the major source of input for each area?	Supplementary: ventral anterior nucleus (VA) relay from basal ganglia Premotor: ventrolateral nucleus (VL) relay primarily from cerebellum
Where is the primary motor cortex located?	Precentral gyrus
What is the name of the pyramidal neurons of primary motor cortex giving rise to the largest axons of the corticospinal tract?	Betz cells
Describe the path of the lateral corticospinal tract:	1. Cortex 2. Corona radiata 3. Posterior limb of internal capsule 4. Cerebral peduncles 5. Longitudinal fibers of the pons 6. Medullary pyramids 7. Lateral column of spinal cord 8. Synapse in ventral horn
Where does the lateral corticospinal tract decussate?	Caudal medulla
Lesion of the corticospinal tract below the caudal medulla will cause hemiparesis of which side of the body?	Ipsilateral
Lesion of the corticospinal tract above the caudal medulla will cause hemiparesis of which side of the body?	Contralateral
What is the name of the uncrossed portion of the corticospinal tract?	Ventral corticospinal tract

Which muscle groups are controlled by the ventral corticospinal tract?	Axial and proximal
What is the name of the tract that innervates motor nuclei of the brainstem?	Corticobulbar
What other structures are innervated by the corticobulbar tract?	Red nucleus and reticular formation
Muscles on which side of the face are controlled by the corticobulbar tract?	The upper face receives bilateral cortical input, while the lower face receives contralateral input.
How is a central lesion differentiated from a peripheral facial palsy?	Peripheral facial lesions prevent forehead wrinkling on physical examination.
Which cranial nerve motor nuclei are not innervated by the corticobulbar tract?	Extraoculars (III, IV, VI)
Which extrapyramidal system is involved in control of extraocular muscles via input from the frontal eye fields (FEF)?	Basal ganglia
In which region of the primary motor cortex does the corticobulbar tract originate?	Lateral region—near the Sylvian fissure
Which region of the cortex controls the muscles of the most inferior extremities?	Medial region—near the sagittal fissure
Which portions of the internal capsule contain fibers of the corticospinal and corticobulbar tracts, respectively?	Corticospinal: posterior limb Corticobulbar: genu and posterior limb
Describe the somatotopic organization of the corticospinal and corticobulbar tracts as they traverse the cerebral peduncle:	Trunk and extremities: lateral Face: medial
What is the term for the exaggerated reflex response and increased resistance to muscle stretch associated with upper motor neuron lesions?	Spasticity
What is the term used to describe repetition of reflex contractions?	Clonus
What is the term used to describe the rigidity associated with upper motor neuron lesions in which resistance increases in a velocity-dependent manner followed by a decreased resistance to passive stretch?	Clasp knife rigidity

What abnormal reflex is associated with upper motor neuron lesions?	Babinski or plantar reflex
Describe a positive Babinski sign:	Upgoing great toe Fanning of other toes
In what population is a positive Babinski considered normal?	Infants up to 1 year of age
Why do infants have a positive Babinski reflex?	Incomplete myelination of the corticospinal tract
What is the mechanism of underlying upper motor neuron signs?	Loss of descending inhibition
What are the signs of upper motor neuron disease?	Spasticity Clasp knife rigidity Babinski sign Clonus

Which type of motor neuron lesion is associated with the following signs:

Affects muscle groups rather than individual muscles	Upper motor neuron
Atrophy	Lower motor neuron
Spasticity	Upper motor neuron
Reduced deep tendon reflexes (DTR)	Lower motor neuron
Babinski sign	Upper motor neuron
Fasciculations	Lower motor neuron
Abnormal nerve conduction and electromyography (EMG)	Lower motor neuron
What is the term used to describe the period of flaccid paralysis that precedes spasticity following corticospinal lesions?	Spinal shock
What is the term used to describe the inability to execute complex motor tasks in the absence of weakness, ataxia, or sensory loss?	Apraxia
Which region of the cortex is responsible for initiation of complex motor tasks?	Frontal lobes
Describe decorticate posturing seen in some comatose patients:	Arms and wrists flexed against the chest, legs extended

What lesions cause decorticate posturing?	Lesion of the corticospinal tract above the red nucleus
What descending motor tracts are likely responsible for decorticate posturing?	Rubrospinal, vestibulospinal, and reticulospinal
Describe decerebrate posturing:	Arms and legs extended
What lesions are associated with degeneration to decerebrate posturing?	Spreading of the lesion below the red nucleus
What descending motor tract originates in the red nucleus?	Rubrospinal tract
Where does the rubrospinal tract decussate?	Midbrain
Describe the regulation of muscle tone for which the rubrospinal tract is responsible:	Flexor tone of the upper extremities
Name the indirect descending motor pathways:	Rubrospinal Reticulospinal Vestibulospinal Tectospinal

Table 7.4 Descending Motor Pathways

Tract	Origin	Decussation	Function
Lateral Corticospinal	Motor cortex	Caudal medulla	Limb muscle control
Ventral Corticospinal	Motor cortex	Ipsilateral	Axial muscle control (cervical region)
Corticobulbar	Motor cortex	Mostly bilateral	Cranial muscle control
Rubrospinal	Red nucleus	Midbrain	Upper limb flexor tone
Lateral Vestibulospinal	Lateral Vestibular Nucleus	Ipsilateral	Balance and posture
Medial Vestibulospinal	Medial Vestibular Nucleus	Bilateral	Head position
Reticulospinal	Reticular Formation	Ipsilateral	Automatic movements (walking)
Tectospinal	Superior Colliculus	Midbrain	Match neck movements with eye movements

BASAL GANGLIA

Which motor region of the brain is typically referred to when using the term extrapyramidal?	Basal ganglia
In which functions of motor control are the basal ganglia involved?	Postural control, initiation, sequencing, and modulation
Which structures make up the basal ganglia?	Caudate nucleus Putamen Globus pallidus Substantia nigra Subthalamic nucleus
What are the thalamic targets of efferents from the basal ganglia?	VL, VA, and intralaminar nuclei
What is the ultimate cortical target of basal ganglia information from the thalamus?	Premotor cortex
What are the differences between the direct and indirect pathways?	Type of striatal dopamine transmission (direct: D1, indirect: D2) (see Fig. 7.1.) Indirect pathway includes globus externa and subthalamic nucleus.
Which pathway aids in execution of cortically activated movements?	Direct pathway
Which pathway prevents unintended movements?	Indirect pathway
Which disease is caused by the loss of dopaminergic neurons in the substantia nigra pars compacta?	Parkinson disease
What designer drug contaminant is metabolized into a toxic compound causing a Parkinson-like syndrome?	1-Methyl-4-phenyl-1,2,3,6-tetrahydropyridine (MPTP)—a meperidine analog
What other drugs are capable of causing Parkinson-like syndromes?	Reserpine, phenothiazines, and haloperidol

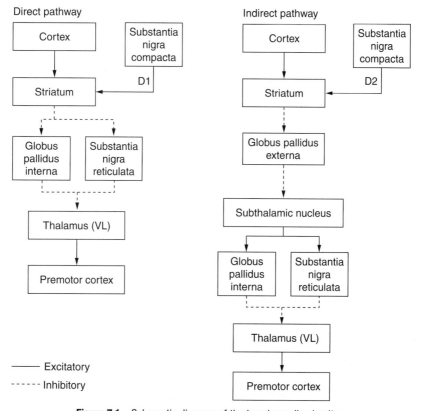

Figure 7.1 Schematic diagram of the basal ganglia circuitry.

Why isn't dopamine used to treat Parkinson disease?

1. Does not cross the blood-brain barrier
2. Systemic effects

What drug is used as dopamine replacement therapy in Parkinson disease?

L-DOPA—a dopamine precursor

What drug is given to prevent peripheral metabolism of L-DOPA by decarboxylases?

Carbidopa
(see Chap. 18)

What other types of drugs are used in the treatment of Parkinson disease?

Catechol-O-methyltransferase (COMT) inhibitors
Monoamine oxidase (MAO) inhibitors
Dopamine agonists

What is the mechanism of action for COMT and MAO inhibitors?

Inhibition of dopamine breakdown

What surgical interventions have shown success in treating Parkinson disease?

Pallidotomy and deep brain stimulation (DBS) of the subthalamic nucleus

What is the pathologic hallmark of Parkinson disease?

Lewy bodies containing α-synuclein

What are the symptoms of Parkinson disease?

Festinating gait

Cogwheel rigidity

Bradykinesia

Hypokinesia

Masked facies

Resting tremor (pill rolling)

What treatments are effective at suppressing essential tremor?

Alcohol, beta-blockers, and some antiepileptic drugs

What is the name of the disease, also known as hepatolenticular degeneration, which causes rigidity and tremor in addition to liver disease?

Wilson disease

What region of the basal ganglia is affected in Wilson disease?

Putamen

What is the defect responsible for Wilson disease?

Deficiency of ceruloplasmin—a copper-binding protein

What is the pathognomonic eye finding in Wilson disease?

Kayser-Fleischer rings (copper deposits)

What is the term used to describe flexion of the hands following dorsiflexion?

Asterixis

In what condition is asterixis commonly seen?

Hepatic encephalopathy

What is the term used to describe the arrhythmic, jerky movements associated with some forms of basal ganglia disease?

Chorea

Which conditions have chorea as a component?

Huntington disease, benign hereditary chorea, senile chorea, and Sydenham chorea

Sydenham chorea is associated with infection by what organism?

Streptococcus pyogenes—one of the Jones criteria for rheumatic fever

What basal ganglia structures are affected by Huntington disease?

Striatum, particularly caudate nucleus (see Chap. 14)

What is the term used to describe the inability to sustain posture, with writhing movements of the hands and face that flow together, seen with fetal hemolysis (kernicterus)?	Athetosis
How is cognitive function affected in kernicterus?	Cognition is relatively spared.
What movement disorder, usually involving the face and mouth, is caused by use of antipsychotics?	Tardive dyskinesia
What other conditions are associated with athetosis?	Fetal hypoxia, hepatic encephalopathy, Huntington disease, Wilson disease, Hallervorden-Spatz disease, and Leigh disease
Leigh disease is due to a genetic disease of which organelle?	Mitochondria (see Chap. 15)
What is the term used to describe the unilateral uncontrollable flinging of limbs?	Hemiballismus
What structure is involved in lesions causing hemiballismus?	Subthalamic nucleus
What disorder causes unnatural posturing due to simultaneous contraction of opposing muscles?	Dystonia
What is the gene product of the DYT1 gene associated with the severe form of this disease seen in Ashkenazi Jews?	Torsin A
What treatment is used for idiopathic focal dystonias seen in frequently used muscles?	Botulinum toxin injections
What are the symptoms of Gilles de Tourette syndrome (GTS)?	Motor and vocal tics, including sniffing, snorting, and vocalizations
What is the gender predominance of GTS?	Men:women = 3:1
What is the term used to describe involuntary cursing that can be seen in GTS?	Coprolalia
What is the prognosis for GTS tics?	Nearly half subside by early adulthood, some go into remission, while still others persist

What other neuropsychiatric disorders are associated with GTS?	Obsessive compulsive disorder and attention-deficit hyperactivity disorder (ADHD)
What treatments are available for GTS?	First-line agents include clonidine and guanfacine; others include Haldol and risperidone

CEREBELLUM

What functions are associated with the cerebellum?	Coordination of skilled movements including the eyes. Control of posture and gait. Equilibrium. Regulation of muscle tone. Motor learning. Many sources describe one of the major functions of the cerebellum as comparing what the cortex wants to do with what the body is actually doing and fixing errors.
In which portion of the skull does the cerebellum reside?	Posterior cranial fossa
What is the name of the thick dural separation between the cerebellum and cerebral cortex?	Tentorium cerebelli
What is the term used for gyri of the cerebellar cortex, because of their leaf-like appearance on cross section?	Folia
What are the three lobes of the cerebellar cortex?	1. Anterior lobe 2. Posterior lobe 3. Flocculonodular lobe
Which functions are associated with each of the following regions of the cerebellum:	
Flocculonodular lobe	Balance and eye movements
Anterior lobe	Limb movements and postural tone
Posterior lobe	Coordination and motor planning
What are the three medial to lateral divisions of the anterior and posterior lobes?	1. Vermis 2. Intermediate regions (known as paravermis) 3. Lateral hemispheres

What neurons provide the major efferent projection from the cerebellar cortex?	Purkinje cells
On what structures do Purkinje cells synapse?	Deep cerebellar nuclei
What are the names of the deep nuclei from medial to lateral?	Fastigial nucleus, globose and emboliform nuclei (known as interposed nuclei), and dentate nucleus

Table 7.5 Cerebellar Peduncles

Peduncle	Fiber Direction	Alternate Name
Superior cerebellar peduncle (SCP)	Mostly efferent	Brachium conjunctivum
Middle cerebellar peduncle (MCP)	Afferent only	Brachium pontis
Inferior cerebellar peduncle (ICP)	Both	Restiform body

What afferent projections pass through the SCP?	Ventral and rostral spinocerebellar tracts
What are the functional divisions of the cerebellum?	Vestibulocerebellum, spinocerebellum, and cerebrocerebellum
To which regions of the cerebellar cortex do the following functional divisions correspond:	
Vestibulocerebellum	Flocculonodular lobe
Spinocerebellum	Vermis and paravermis
Cerebrocerebellum	Lateral hemispheres
To what thalamic nucleus do the deep cerebellar nuclei project?	VL nucleus
Which types of sensory input project to the flocculonodular lobe?	Vestibular and visual input
To which brainstem nuclei does the flocculonodular lobe project?	Vestibular nuclei

Table 7.6 Functional Divisions of the Cerebellum

Functional Division	Input	Anatomic Location	Deep Nucleus	Function
Vestibulocerebellum	Vestibular system	Flocculonodular	—	Regulate balance and eye movement
Spinocerebellum	Spinocerebellar Vestibular Visual Auditory	Vermis Paravermis	Fastigial Interposed	Regulate axial musculature (posture) Regulate limb musculature
Cerebrocerebellum	Cerebral cortex via the pontine nuclei	Lateral hemispheres	Dentate	Motor planning

Table 7.7 Efferent Cerebellar Pathways

	Efferent Projection	Relay	Target	Affected Tract
Flocculonodular lobe	ICP	—	Vestibular nuclei	Vestibulospinal tract Extraoculars (MLF)
Fastigial	ICP	—	Vestibular nuclei	Vestibulospinal tracts
	ICP	—	Reticular formation	Reticulospinal tract
	SCP	VL	Motor cortex	Ventral corticospinal tract
Interposed	SCP	—	Red nucleus	Rubrospinal tract
	SCP	VL	Motor cortex	Lateral corticospinal tract
Dentate	SCP	—	Red nucleus	Inferior olivary nucleus
	SCP	VL	Motor cortex	Motor tracts

Table 7.8 Pathways of the Cerebellum

Input	Functional Division	Anatomic Region	Deep Nucleus	Efferent Projection	Relay	Target	Modulates
Vestibular	Vestibulocerebellum	Flocculonodular lobe	—	ICP	—	Vestibular nuclei	Medial vestibulospinal tracts and extraoculars
Spinocerebellar Vestibular Visual Auditory	Spinocerebellum	Vermis	Fastigial	ICP ... SCP	— ... VL	Vestibular nuclei ... Reticular formation ... Motor cortex	Vestibulospinal tract ... Reticulospinal tract ... Ventral corticospinal tract
Spinocerebellar	Spinocerebellum	Paravermis	Interposed	SCP ... SCP	— ... VL	Red nucleus ... Motor cortex	Rubrospinal tract ... Lateral corticospinal tract
Motor cortex Sensory cortex	Cerebrocerebellum	Lateral hemispheres	Dentate	SCP ... SCP	— ... VL	Red nucleus ... Motor cortex	Inferior olivary nucleus ... Motor tracts

110

Which descending motor tracts are affected by the fastigial nucleus?	Ventral corticospinal, vestibulospinal, and reticulospinal tracts
Through which peduncle do the dentate, emboliform, and globose nuclei project to the thalamus?	SCP
Through which peduncle do the crossed projections from the pontine nuclei reach the cerebellar cortex?	MCP
Which side of the body do lesions of the cerebellum generally affect?	Ipsilateral
Why are ipsilateral limb movements affected?	Cerebellar efferent projections to VL and the red nucleus decussate in the SCP. This offsets the crossing of corticopontocerebellar fibers, as well as the crossing of the lateral corticospinal and rubrospinal tracts. This phenomenon is sometimes referred to as the "double cross."
How are the corticopontocerebellar fibers believed to help the cerebellum coordinate limb movements?	Comparison between desired movement and actual limb trajectories
What are the layers of the cerebellar cortex and corresponding cell types?	Molecular layer: stellate and basket cells (inhibitory interneurons) Purkinje cell layer: Purkinje cells (inhibitory efferent) Granule cell layer: granule cells (excitatory) and Golgi interneurons (inhibitory)
What is the name of the predominant afferent fibers from the spinocerebellar tract, pons, and vestibular system?	Mossy fibers
On which cell types do mossy fibers of the cerebellum synapse?	Granule and Golgi cells
What is the name of the excitatory fibers from the granule cells to the Purkinje cells?	Parallel fibers
What is the name of the fibers from the inferior olivary nucleus?	Climbing fibers
Where do the climbing fibers synapse?	Directly onto the Purkinje cells and deep cerebellar nuclei

What term is used to describe the inability to perform rapidly alternating movements?	Dysdiadochokinesia
What term is used to describe the fragmentation of motor sequences seen in cerebellar lesions?	Decomposition
How would one test for "loss of check?"	Quickly release downward resistance on a patient's outstretched arm—patient will nearly hit their own face (known as Stewart-Holmes sign)
What are the clinical features of cerebellar lesions?	Ataxia Dysdiadochokinesia Decomposition Loss of check Intention tremor Dysmetria Dysfunction of equilibrium and gait Decreased muscle tone Nystagmus Scanning speech Dysarthria
What problems are seen with the following specific cerebellar lesions:	
Lesion of the vermis	Poor balance and broad-based gait
Lesion of the flocculonodular lobe	Dizziness, vomiting, vertigo, and nystagmus
Abuse of what substance can lead to signs of vermal degeneration?	Alcohol
Which tests can be used to examine dysmetria and intention tremor?	Finger-to-nose and heel-to-shin
Which test can be used to examine dysdiadochokinesia?	Rapidly alternating hand pronation/supination or finger-to-thumb tapping
Which test should not be confused as a cerebellar sign?	Romberg sign
What does a positive Romberg sign indicate?	Proprioceptive dysfunction (Dorsal columns)

What disease involves peripheral demyelination with intact sensation, but severe ataxia and intention tremor due to spinocerebellar damage?

Miller-Fisher syndrome

Miller-Fisher syndrome is thought to be a variant of what peripheral demyelinating disease?

Guillain-Barre
(see Chap. 12)

CLINICAL VIGNETTES

Make the diagnosis for the following patients:

A 58-year-old man with a history of HTN, hyperlipidemia, and recent ischemic stroke presents with violent flailing of his arms and legs on the left side of his body. Imaging suggests lesion in the region of the right subthalamic nucleus and surrounding white matter.

Hemiballismus

A 60-year-old woman with no prior medical history complains of gradual onset of a tremor beginning in her right hand that over time also affected her left hand. She has noticed muscle aches with increasing frequency, finds it hard to initiate movements, and feels tired most of the time. Physical examination reveals cogwheel rigidity to passive resistance and paucity of facial expression. She has a resting tremor in her hands with a frequency of about 5 Hz. Her gait involves short strides and very little arm swing. Routine labs and imaging studies are unremarkable.

Parkinson disease

A 45-year-old man with a history of HTN complains of aberrant limb movement and declining intellectual capacity. He has started noticing involuntary movements of his hands. His wife reports that he behaves differently lately, acting impulsively, at times depressed, and has become antisocial. His father died after a 15 year struggle with dementia and movement disorder. Physical examination reveals twitching in his hands and face. MRI of the brain reveals atrophy of the caudate nucleus and enlarged lateral ventricles. Following appropriate pretest counseling, genetic testing reveals CAG expansion in a gene on the short arm chromosome 4.

Huntington disease

A 51-year-old man with a long history of schizophrenia and antipsychotic medication use presents with peculiar writhing movements of his tongue and facial muscles. On physical examination, irregular movements of the tongue and jaw occur at varied intervals. The patient has no family history of movement disorders including Huntington disease or dystonia. Blood tests reveal normal copper and ceruloplasmin levels. Brain imaging reveals only normal findings.

Tardive dyskinesia

A 24-year-old woman presents with jerking and writhing movements and recent yellowing of her skin. She reports that a close relative with similar symptoms died from liver failure at the age of 35. Blood tests show elevated liver enzymes, elevated copper, and low ceruloplasmin; while an MRI shows basal ganglia damage. Eye examination reveals greenish brown rings.

Wilson disease

CHAPTER 8

ANS and Hypothalamus

AUTONOMIC NERVOUS SYSTEM

What does the autonomic nervous system (ANS) control?	Smooth muscle Cardiac function Exocrine glands
What makes the ANS different from the peripheral nervous system?	Motor neurons outside central nervous system (CNS) Nonvoluntary (mostly subconscious) No specialized pre- or postsynaptic regions More diffuse control
In general, how is information transferred from CNS through the ANS?	CNS → ganglion → effector
Generally, how many neurons are involved in the pathway of ANS information from CNS?	Two neurons: preganglionic neuron and postganglionic neuron
Which sympathetic innervation does not involve a postganglionic projection?	Adrenal medulla
What are the three divisions of the ANS and their roles?	1. Sympathetic: fight/flight/fright 2. Parasympathetic: maintain normal body conditions 3. Enteric: gastrointestinal (GI) digestive reflexes
What is another name for the sympathetic nervous system?	Thoracolumbar
What is another name for the parasympathetic nervous system?	Craniosacral
Describe the sympathetic preganglionic axons?	B fibers: slow conducting, myelinated, small diameter

How are postganglionic axons of the sympathetic system different from preganglionic axons? | Unmyelinated, C fibers

Where are the sympathetic ganglia located? | Sympathetic chain—alongside the vertebral column and preaortic ganglia

At what spinal levels do preganglionic neurons of the sympathetic system originate? | T1-L3

What is the name of the structure/nucleus from which preganglionic sympathetic neurons originate? | Intermediolateral cell column

What target organs are innervated bilaterally? | Intestines and pelvic viscera

What is the ratio of pre- to postganglionic fibers of the sympathetic system? | 1:10

What is the ratio of pre- to postganglionic fibers in the parasympathetic system? | 1:3

Identify the labeled structures in Fig. 8.1:

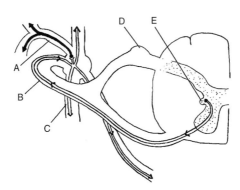

Figure 8.1   Wiring diagram of the sympathetic nervous system.

A   Gray ramus
B   White ramus
C   Sympathetic trunk

D   Dorsal root ganglion
E   Intermediolateral cell column

Name the preganglionic fibers that project from the intermediolateral cell column to the ganglia of the sympathetic chain: | White rami

How are white rami different from gray rami? | White rami are preganglionic and myelinated

Where do axons that make up the white rami leave the spinal cord? | Ventral root

What are the ganglia of the sympathetic trunk called?	Paravertebral
To what ganglia do the splanchnic nerves project?	Prevertebral (aka collateral)
What sympathetic ganglion supplies most of the head?	Superior cervical (SCG)
What constitutes the SCG?	Fused ganglia of C1-C4
What is the pathway of sympathetic input to the dilator pupillae?	1. Hypothalamus 2. Ciliospinal center of Budge (T1/T2 level) 3. SCG 4. Follow internal carotid to cavernous sinus 5. Nasociliary and long ciliary nerves (CN V) or caroticotympanic nerves 6. Orbit: innervating iris dilator and Müller muscle
In the sympathetic system, what is the major neurotransmitter (NT) of the preganglionic neurons?	Acetylcholine (ACh)
What type of ACh receptor is found at the sympathetic ganglia?	Nicotinic
What is the major NT of the postganglionic sympathetic neurons?	Norepinephrine (NE)
What postganglionic sympathetic innervation uses ACh instead of NE?	Sweat glands
What type of receptor is found at the sweat glands?	Muscarinic ACh receptor
Where is dopamine involved in the sympathetic system?	Inhibitory interneurons in ganglia (small intensely fluorescent [SIF] cells)
What type of adrenergic receptor (AR) controls sympathetic effect on cutaneous and splanchnic arteries and arterioles?	Alpha
What is the effect of alpha-receptor stimulation of these vessels?	Constriction
What type of AR controls the effect of the sympathetic system on skeletal muscle vasculature?	Beta

What is the effect of beta-receptor stimulation on skeletal muscle vasculature?	Dilation
What type of AR controls the effect of the sympathetic system on heart musculature?	$Beta_1$
What is the main NT of the parasympathetic system?	Ach
What is the receptor of the preganglionic synapses in the parasympathetic system?	Nicotinic
What is the receptor of the postganglionic synapses in the parasympathetic system?	Muscarinic
What other hormones are involved in some postganglionic parasympathetic fibers?	Vasoactive intestinal peptide (VIP) and nitric oxide (NO)
How is the parasympathetic system anatomically different from the sympathetic system?	1. Location of preganglionic cell origin 2. Ganglia are near the effectors, therefore, have longer preganglionic axons
Where do parasympathetic preganglionic cells originate?	Brainstem and S2-S4 regions of spinal cord

Table 8.1 Cranial Nerve Parasympathetic Innervations

Cranial Nerve	Nucleus	Function
CN III	Edinger-Westphal	Pupil constriction
CN VII	Superior salivatory	Submandibular, sublingual, lacrimal secretion
CN IX	Inferior salivatory	Parotid secretion
CN X	Dorsal motor nucleus Nucleus ambiguus	Viscera of thorax and abdomen Heart, esophagus, lungs

What is the pathway of parasympathetic innervation of the eye?	1. Edinger-Westphal nucleus 2. CN III 3. Ciliary ganglion 4. Short ciliary nerves 5. Sphincter pupillae and ciliary muscle

What are the symptoms of a lesion of the parasympathetic innervation of the eye?	Fixed and dilated pupil (internal ophthalmoplegia), failure to accommodate (cycloplegia)
What ganglion is associated with parasympathetic innervation of the lacrimal gland and nasal and palate mucosa?	Pterygopalatine
By which cranial nerve are the lacrimal gland and nasal and palatal mucosa innervated?	CN VII
Which ganglion is associated with parasympathetic innervation of the submandibular and sublingual glands?	Submandibular
Which ganglion is associated with parasympathetic innervation of the parotid gland?	Otic
Which ganglion is associated with innervation of the SA and AV nodes?	Cardiac ganglia
From which nucleus do the fibers innervating the SA and AV nodes arise?	Nucleus ambiguus, ventrolateral group of neurons
Up to what point in the GI tract does the vagus nerve innervate the abdominal viscera?	Left colic flexure
Where does parasympathetic innervation originate after the left colic flexure?	Sacral spine
Through what nerves does the parasympathetic innervation to the lower GI tract travel?	Pelvic splanchnic nerves
What are the functions of the sacral division of the parasympathetic nervous system?	Micturition Defecation Sexual function
How is the enteric system different from the rest of the ANS?	Relatively independent of CNS
Which parts of the GI specifically are most autonomous?	Small and large intestines

Table 8.2 Autonomic Innervations

Structure	Sympathetic	Parasympathetic
Eye		
Radial muscle of iris	Mydriasis	
Circular muscle of iris		Miosis
Ciliary muscle		Contracts to focus vision
Müller muscle	Contracts to retract eyelid	
Lacrimal gland		Secretion
Salivary glands	Viscous secretion	Watery secretion
Sweat glands	Stimulate	
Heart		
SA node	Accelerates	Decelerates
AV node	Increases velocity of conduction	Decreases velocity
Contractility	Increases	Decreases (atria)
Vascular smooth muscle		
Skin and splanchnic vessels	Contracts	
Skeletal vessels	Relaxes	
Bronchiolar smooth muscle	Relaxes	Contracts
GI tract		
Smooth muscle		
Walls	Relaxes	Contracts
Sphincters	Contracts	Relaxes
Secretion and motility	Decreases	Increases
Adrenal medulla	Secrete catecholamines	
Liver	Gluconeogenesis and glycogenolysis	
Adipocytes	Lipolysis	
Kidney	Release renin	
GU tract smooth muscle		
Bladder wall		Contracts
Sphincter	Contracts	Relaxes
Penis and seminal vesicles	Ejaculation	Erection
Skin		
Pilomotor smooth muscle	Contracts	
Sweat glands	Thermoregulation (muscarinic) Stress activated (α-AR)	

How many neurons are in the enteric nervous system (ENS)?	Approximately same number as in spinal cord, 80 to 100 million
What are the excitatory NTs of the ENS?	ACh and substance P
What are the inhibitory NTs of the ENS motor neurons?	Dynorphin and VIP
Name the cell body plexuses of the enteric system (both names):	Myenteric or Auerbach and submucosal or Meissner
Where are the cell body plexuses of the enteric system located?	Myenteric: between outer and longitudinal and inner circular muscles Submucosal: between circular muscle and mucosa
What are the general functions of the myenteric and submucosal plexuses?	Myenteric: motility Submucosal: secretion

PATHOLOGY

What is the most common and most overlooked early symptom of autonomic dysfunction?	Impotence
What is the most common disabling feature of autonomic dysfunction?	Orthostatic hypotension
What is an autonomic cause of excess HCl production in peptic ulcer disease?	Increased parasympathetic tone
What congenital disease is characterized by dilation and hypertrophy of the colon?	Hirschsprung disease (congenital aganglionic megacolon)
What is the cause of Hirschsprung disease?	Failure of migration of neural crest cells
What are the presenting symptoms of Hirschsprung disease?	Failure to pass meconium within 48 hours of birth Bowel obstruction with bilious vomiting Poor feeding/failure to thrive Abdominal distention

What acquired disease resembles Hirschsprung disease? — Chagas disease

What are the symptoms of chronic Chagas disease? — Megacolon, megaesophagus, arrhythmias

How is the ANS affected by Chagas disease? — Autoimmune destruction of autonomic nerves after *Trypanosoma cruzi* infection

What syndrome causes ptosis, miosis, hemihydrosis, enopthalmos, and flushing? — Horner syndrome

What is the cause of Horner syndrome? — Lesion of sympathetic input to eye anywhere along chain

What is the hallmark of central (preganglionic) Horner syndrome? — Dilated iris

What would you see in postganglionic Horner syndrome? — Nondilated iris

The effect of Horner syndrome on melanocytes in the iris can lead to what eye finding in children with congenital disease or acquired Horner prior to age 2? — Heterochromia: one eye lighter than the other

What tumor of lung origin can cause Horner syndrome? — Pancoast tumor

What syndrome is a combination of Parkinsonism and autonomic dysfunction? — Shy-Drager syndrome

What are the autonomic symptoms of Shy-Drager syndrome? — Orthostatic hypotension, secretion disturbances, impotence, pupil abnormalities

What is the cause of the sympathetic dysfunction in Shy-Drager syndrome? — Degeneration of intermediolateral neurons

What is Raynaud phenomenon? — Reversible ischemia of peripheral arterioles, most commonly due to cold or stress

What is a treatment for Raynaud disease involving the ANS? — Preganglionic sympathectomy

What disease is characterized by abnormal sweating, orthostatic hypotension, inadequate muscle tone in GI, absence of lingual fungiform papillae, and progressive sensory loss?	Familial dysautonomia (Riley-Day syndrome)
What is the mode of inheritance of familial dysautonomia?	Autosomal recessive
What ethnic group does familial dysautonomia mostly affect?	Ashkenazi Jews
What is the cause of familial dysautonomia?	Loss of autonomic and sensory ganglia neurons

HYPOTHALAMUS

What is the main function of the hypothalamus?	Maintain homeostasis
What systems does the hypothalamus control?	ANS Endocrine system Limbic system
Where is the hypothalamus located?	Floor and ventral walls of the anterior third ventricle
Which part of the hypothalamus stimulates the parasympathetic division of the ANS?	Anterior
Which part of the hypothalamus stimulates the sympathetic division of the ANS?	Posterior
What are the major functional divisions of the hypothalamus?	Lateral and medial areas
Which nuclei lie in the lateral hypothalamic area?	Lateral preoptic nucleus, lateral hypothalamic nucleus (LHN)
What is the function of the LHN?	Feeding center
What is the consequence of a lesion in the LHN?	Anorexia

What are the four regions of the medial hypothalamic area?

(anterior → posterior)
1. Preoptic
2. Supraoptic
3. Tuberal
4. Mammillary

What nucleus in the preoptic region contains the sexually dimorphic nucleus?

Medial preoptic nucleus

What is the function of the medial preoptic nucleus?

Regulate release of gonadotropic hormones from pituitary

What are the nuclei of the supraoptic region?

Suprachiasmatic, anterior, paraventricular, supraoptic

What is the function of the suprachiasmatic nucleus?

Circadian rhythm

What is the function of the anterior nucleus?

Temperature regulation

What is the symptom of a lesion in the anterior nucleus?

Hyperthermia

What is the homeostatic role of the paraventricular nucleus (PVN)?

Regulate water balance

How does PVN regulate water balance?

Synthesis and secretion of antidiuretic hormone (ADH) and corticotropin-releasing hormone (CRH)

What stimulates the release of ADH?

Decreased blood volume and increased osmolality

What is the effect of ADH secretion?

Water retention by kidneys

What is the molecular mechanism of ADH action on the kidney?

Insertion of aquaporins into the distal and collecting tubules of the nephron

What else do the neurons of the PVN make?

Oxytocin

What are the primary functions of oxytocin?

Lactation and uterine contraction

What is the result of a lesion in the PVN?

Diabetes insipidus

What is the function of the supraoptic nucleus?

Synthesize ADH and oxytocin

Where do the products synthesized by the supraoptic nucleus get delivered?	Posterior pituitary (neurohypophysis)
How do ADH and oxytocin synthesized by the supraoptic nucleus get to the posterior pituitary?	Supraopticohypophyseal tract and portal system
What are the nuclei of the tuberal region?	Dorsomedial, ventromedial, and arcuate nuclei
What is the result of stimulation of the dorsomedial nucleus?	Rage
What is the function of the ventromedial nucleus?	Satiety center
What is the result of bilateral lesions in the ventromedial nucleus?	Hyperphagia, obesity, rage
What is the main function of the arcuate nucleus?	Stimulate or inhibit release of hormones from anterior pituitary (adenohypophysis)
How does the arcuate nucleus control the release of the pituitary hormones?	Hypothalamic releasing and inhibitory peptides and dopamine
What are the peptide releasing factors that control pituitary hormones?	Thyrotropin-releasing hormone (TRH), gonadotropin-releasing hormone (GnRH), growth hormone-releasing hormone (GHRH), and CRH
What is the peptide-inhibitory factor that regulates pituitary hormones?	Somatostatin
What does somatostatin inhibit?	Growth hormone
What is the role of dopamine released from the arcuate?	Prolactin inhibitory factor
What is the name of the syndrome due to lack of hypothalamic GnRH associated with hypogonadism and anosmia, among other things?	Kallmann syndrome
To what peptide released from adipose tissue is the arcuate nucleus responsive?	Leptin

What are the molecular effects of leptin on the arcuate nucleus?

Decreased production of neuropeptide Y (NPY) and agouti-related peptide (AgRP)

Increased proopiomelanocortin (POMC)

What are the effects of leptin (through POMC, NPY, and AGRP) on the paraventricular and lateral hypothalamic nuclei?

Inhibits food intake and increases energy expenditure

What are the nuclei of the mammillary region?

Mammillary bodies and posterior nucleus

What is the function of the posterior nucleus?

Thermal regulation

What is the symptom of a lesion in the posterior nucleus?

Poikilothermia

What is the syndrome characterized by a rapid rise in body temperature >40°C, rigidity, and autonomic dysregulation?

Malignant hyperthermia

What are some pharmacologic causes of malignant hyperthermia?

Antipsychotics (neuroleptics), inhalational anesthetics, succinylcholine

What muscle relaxer is effective in treating malignant hyperthermia?

Dantrolene

What are the symptoms of hypothalamic syndrome?

Adiposity, diabetes insipidus, somnolence, lack of temperature regulation

What causes hypothalamic syndrome?

Pressure on the hypothalamus (eg, tumor, sarcoidosis, and inflammation)

Projections from the mammillary bodies are a part of what circuit or system?

Papez circuit–limbic system

Where does information from the mammillary nuclei project in the Papez circuit?

Anterior nucleus of the thalamus

What is the limbic system?

Structures of the brain involved in memory, emotion, and behavior

| What is the Papez circuit? | Circuit that connects major limbic structures for memory storage (see Fig. 8.2) |

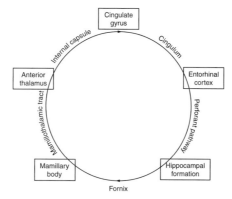

Figure 8.2 Schematic diagram of the Papez circuit.

| What other part of the brain is closely associated with the limbic system, though it is not depicted in the Papez circuit? | Amygdala |

| What emotion is associated with the amygdala? | Fear |

| What results from stimulation of the amygdala in primates? | Feeding, aggressive behavior |

| From what structures does the amygdala receive input? | Olfactory tract, hypothalamus, hippocampus, and limbic and association cortices |

| Where does the amygdala send input? | Hypothalamus, brainstem, and limbic and association cortices |

| In what disorder do you see lesions of the mammillary bodies? | Wernicke encephalopathy |

| What is the cause of Wernicke encephalopathy? | Thiamine (B_1) deficiency |

| What is the main population affected by Wernicke encephalopathy? | Alcoholics |

| What are the characteristic symptoms of Wernicke encephalopathy? | Ocular palsy, ataxic gait, confusion, drowsiness |

What other syndrome is often seen with Wernicke encephalopathy?	Korsakoff syndrome
What are the symptoms of Korsakoff syndrome?	Amnesia and confabulation
How is it different from Wernicke encephalopathy?	Irreversible
Where is the lesion responsible for Korsakoff syndrome?	Mediodorsal thalamus
What is the treatment for Wernicke encephalopathy?	Thiamine
What common clinical intervention can precipitate Wernicke encephalopathy in a thiamine deficient patient?	Intravenous dextrose administration

CLINICAL VIGNETTES

Make the diagnosis for the following patients:

A 1-year-old female of Ashkenazi Jewish descent is brought in by her parents who complain that she has problems with hearing and vision, is moody, and prone to tantrums, but does not have tears when she cries. They have also noticed that she sweats excessively. On physical examination, she is hyporeflexive, orthostatic, insensitive to pain, and exhibits abnormal sweating. She lacks fungiform papillae on her tongue. Fluorescein reveals corneal ulceration. A genetic diagnosis is made based on the presence of the *IKBKAP* mutation.

> Familial dysautonomia (Riley-Day syndrome)

A 57-year-old female smoker with a 55-pack-year history is currently being treated for squamous cell carcinoma. She complains of intermittent pain in her left shoulder and along the forearm, as well as weakness in her hand. On examining the patient, you notice that her left pupil is smaller than her right. Pupillary reflex is intact in the right eye. She also has ptosis of her left eyelid. Chest CT reveals a large tumor in the left lung apex.

> Horner syndrome secondary to Pancoast tumor

An 18-year-old female complains of episodic, sometimes painful cyanosis of the fingers, usually in response to cold or stress. Physical examination is negative for sclerodactyly and ulcers of the fingers. Blood tests are negative for autoantibodies. There are no signs or history of collagen-vascular disease, vasculitis, or paraneoplastic etiology.

> Raynaud phenomenon (primary)

A newborn male infant is brought to your office for evaluation of distended abdomen and failure to thrive. The parents report that the infant does not have regular bowel movements, is not feeding well, and occasionally vomits yellow-green colored fluid. Plain abdominal films show distended bowel loops; barium enema demonstrates dilation of the proximal colon with distal narrowing. Rectal biopsy confirms the absence of ganglion cells in this distal segment of bowel.

Hirschsprung disease

A 24-year-old male with a recent history of transsphenoidal surgery to remove a large prolactinoma complains of excessive urination, including waking up from sleep to urinate. In addition, he reports constant thirst. Physical examination is unremarkable. Blood tests reveal normal glucose level. Urine specific gravity is reported at 1.004. Urine osmolality of 150 mOsm/kg with a plasma osmolality of 290 mOsm/kg. Water deprivation testing and exogenous antidiuretic hormone (ADH) confirm the suspected diagnosis.

Central diabetes insipidus

CHAPTER 9

Vascular and Traumatic Injury

VASCULAR ANATOMY

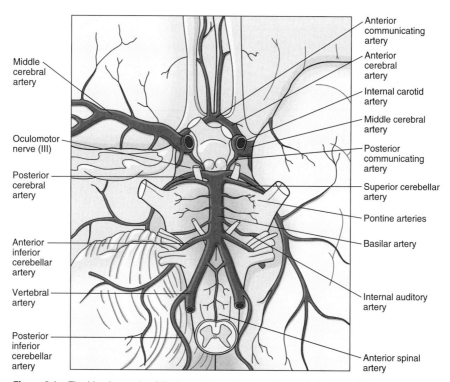

Figure 9.1 The blood vessels of the brain. (Reproduced with permission from Kandel ER, Schwartz JH, Jessel TM, eds. *Principles of Neural Science.* 4th ed. New York, NY: McGraw-Hill; 2000: 1303.)

What vessels make up the anterior circulation?	Internal carotid arteries and branches
What vessels make up the posterior circulation?	Vertebral arteries and branches
Which of these supplies the brainstem?	Posterior circulation
Which vessels supplying the spinal cord are fed by vertebral arteries?	Anterior spinal artery and posterior spinal arteries (2)
What part of the brain is supplied by the anterior spinal artery?	Caudal medulla

What type of branches from the posterior circulation feed the following regions of the brainstem:

Midline brainstem	Paramedian branches
Lateral brainstem	Short circumferential branches
Dorsolateral and cerebellum	Long circumferential branches

Table 9.1 Vasculature of the Brainstem

Artery	Branch	Structure
Vertebral	Paramedian arteries	Medial medulla
	Posterior inferior cerebellar (PICA)	Lateral medulla
		Caudal cerebellum
Basilar	Paramedian arteries	Medial pons
		Caudal midbrain
	Anterior inferior cerebellar (AICA)	Caudal pons (dorsolateral)
		Middle cerebellum
	Superior cerebellar (SCA)	Rostral pons (dorsolateral)
		Rostral cerebellum
		Inferior colliculi
Posterior cerebral (PCA)	Paramedian arteries	Medial midbrain
	Long circumferential	Superior colliculi

What artery passes through the cavernous sinus?	Internal carotid artery (ICA)
What do the following deep branches of the cerebral segment of the ICA supply:	
Ophthalmic artery	CN II and the retina (via central retinal artery)
Posterior communicating artery (PCoA) supplies	Diencephalon
Anterior choroidal artery	Part of the diencephalon, globus pallidus (interna), amygdala, and internal capsule
What are the major cerebral branches of the ICA?	Anterior cerebral (ACA) and middle cerebral (MCA)
What remaining vessels in the circle of Willis are branches of the ICA?	Anterior communicating artery (ACoA) and PCoA
What two vessels are connected by the ACoA?	1. Left ACA 2. Right ACA
What two vessels are connected by the PCoA?	1. Middle cerebral artery (MCA) 2. PCA

Table 9.2 Vasculature of the Cerebral Cortex

Vessel	Course	Region Supplied
ACA	Curves around the corpus callosum within the sagittal fissure	Dorsomedial frontal and parietal lobes
MCA	Runs within Sylvian fissure	Lateral convexity of the cerebral cortex
PCA	Curves behind the midbrain	Occipital lobe and inferior and medial temporal lobe

Identify the labeled vessels from the
angiogram in Fig. 9.2:

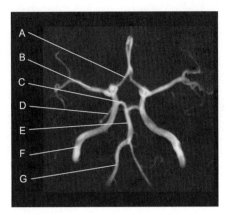

Figure 9.2   Magnetic resonance angiogram of cerebral vasculature.

A   Anterior cerebral artery
B   Middle cerebral artery
C   Posterior communicating artery
D   Posterior cerebral artery

E   Basilar artery
F   Internal carotid artery
G   Vertebral artery

What parts of the central nervous system (CNS) have venous drainage into systemic venous plexuses?	Spinal cord and caudal medulla
What are the low pressure channels into which venous blood from the remainder of the CNS drains?	Dural venous sinuses
Between which layers of the dura are these cerebral venous sinuses found?	Between meningeal and periosteal layers
Name the two dural venous sinuses in the falx cerebri that receive blood from superficial cerebral veins.	1. Superior sagittal sinuses 2. Inferior sagittal sinuses
What sinus is formed by the junction of the deep cerebral vein of Galen with the inferior sagittal sinus?	Straight sinus
What is the name of the place at which the straight sinus and superior sagittal sinus merge?	Confluence of sinuses
From the confluence of sinuses, what is the course of venous blood draining via the internal jugular vein?	1. Transverse sinus 2. Sigmoid sinus 3. Internal jugular vein

In what dural structure that separates the cerebellum from the cerebral cortex are many venous sinuses found?

Tentorium cerebelli

What drains the following structures:

    Pons and rostral medulla

Superior petrosal sinus

    Midbrain, basal ganglia, diencephalons, and deep white matter

Great cerebral vein of Galen

    Cerebellum

Both superior petrosal sinus and vein of Galen

What dural sinus that surrounds the body of the sphenoid bone drains into the inferior and superior petrosal sinuses?

Cavernous sinus

What vein drained by the cavernous sinus contains blood facial vein, and is a potential source of infection from acne?

Ophthalmic vein

What other valveless veins are a potential source of infection in the cavernous sinus?

Emissary veins

CEREBROVASCULAR DISEASE

What type of cell death typically occurs as a result of ischemia?

Necrosis

How long can ischemia persist before permanent damage is likely to occur?

5 minutes

What is an effective method for increasing the amount of time before which permanent ischemic damage occurs?

Lowering body temperature

What are the two types of cerebral infarction?

1. Thrombosis
2. Embolism

Which is more common, a thrombotic or embolic occlusion?

Thrombotic occlusion

What is the name of the infarct caused by the trapping of an object that originated in another location?

Embolic occlusion

What is the major risk factor for thrombotic occlusion?

Atherosclerosis

What is the major source of emboli to the brain?

Cardiac mural thrombi

What are the major risk factors for cardiac mural thrombi?

Myocardial infarct, valvular disease, and atrial fibrillation

What are the two most common sites for thrombotic occlusion?

1. MCA
2. Carotid bifurcation

What is the most common site for embolic occlusion?

MCA

Which type of occlusion is typically associated with a hemorrhagic (red) infarction?

Embolic occlusion

What is the most likely mechanism underlying hemorrhagic infarction?

Reperfusion injury

Which type of occlusion is typically associated with nonhemorrhagic (pale, bland, anemic) infarcts?

Thrombotic occlusion

What is the term used to describe brain regions lying on the border of zones supplied by major cerebral arteries, making them most susceptible to ischemia?

Watershed zones

What is the cause of watershed infarctions?

Inadequate cerebral perfusion due to pump failure

How can you calculate cerebral perfusion pressure (CPP)?

CPP = Mean arterial pressure – ICP
Or if jugular venous pressure > ICP, CPP = Mean arterial – jugular venous

What are some of the more common causes of pump failure that can lead to watershed infarctions?

Myocardial infarction, arrhythmia, pericardial effusion, and pulmonary embolus

What are the two characteristic syndromes of watershed infarction?

1. Visual agnosia and cortical blindness
2. Arm and shoulder paresis

Ischemia of the zone between which two vessels is responsible for visual agnosia?

MCA and PCA

What is the name for infarctions caused by small vessel occlusive disease causing cavitary lesions (lacunae)?

Lacunar strokes

In what type of vessels do lacunar strokes happen?

Deep penetrating arteries

What brain regions are most often involved in lacunar strokes?	Basal ganglia, internal capsule, thalamus, corona radiata, and the pons
What are the five lacunar syndromes?	1. Pure motor 2. Ataxic hemiparesis 3. Dysarthria/clumsy hand 4. Pure sensory 5. Mixed sensorimotor

STROKE SYNDROMES

What artery is occluded if a patient presents with contralateral hemiplegia especially of upper extremities, contralateral hemisensory loss especially of upper extremities, homonymous hemianopia, and aphasia?	Dominant MCA
What area of the brain is affected by an occlusion of the MCA?	Lateral aspect of brain: parietal, frontal, and temporal lobes
What expressive/nonfluent aphasia results from diminished MCA supply to the inferior gyrus of the frontal lobe in the dominant hemisphere?	Broca aphasia
What are the symptoms of Broca aphasia?	The patient speaks slowly and with difficulty, but has good comprehension of speech.
What receptive/fluent aphasia results from occlusion of the MCA supply to the posterior aspect of the dominant superior temporal gyrus?	Wernicke aphasia
What are the symptoms of Wernicke aphasia?	The patient speaks quickly and incoherently with poor comprehension of the spoken language.
What artery is occluded if a patient presents with contralateral hemiplegia, homonymous hemianopsia, contralateral hemisensory deficit, sensory neglect, and apraxia?	Nondominant MCA
What artery is occluded if a patient presents with contralateral hemiplegia especially of the lower extremities, contralateral hemisensory deficit especially of the lower extremities, and urinary incontinence?	ACA

What area of the brain does the ACA supply?	Medial frontal and parietal lobes
What allows for sparing of the macula in a patient with contralateral homonymous hemianopsia resulting from occlusion of the PCA?	Collateral supply from MCA
What term is used to describe the symptom of a shade coming down over the eye when a patient describes a complete or partial transient loss of vision?	Amaurosis fugax
What artery is most likely completely or partially occluded in a patient describing amaurosis fugax?	Ophthalmic artery
What classic embolic syndrome includes ipsilateral blindness (amaurosis fugax), contralateral hemiparalysis, and contralateral hemisensory deficit?	Carotid embolic syndrome
What classic embolic syndrome includes drop attacks, bilateral blindness, confusion, and vertigo?	Vertebrobasilar emboli
What is the name of the syndrome in a patient who presents with contralateral hemisensory deficit of body, ipsilateral hemisensory deficit of face, dysmetria, ataxia, ipsilateral Horner syndrome, aspiration, vertigo, and double vision resulting from PICA occlusion?	Lateral medullary syndrome(Wallenberg)
What artery is most likely occluded in a patient with Wallenberg syndrome?	Vertebral artery, causing damage in the area supplied by PICA
What is the name of the syndrome characterized by ipsilateral eye "down and out," mydriasis, and contralateral paralysis of extremities, face, and tongue?	Weber syndrome (see Table 3.5)
What area of the brainstem is affected in Weber syndrome?	Ventral midbrain
What arteries are most likely occluded in Weber syndrome?	Paramedian perforating arteries of the basilar artery or PCA

INTRACRANIAL HEMORRHAGE

What are the two types of nontraumatic brain hemorrhages?	1. Intracerebral 2. Subarachnoid
What is the major risk factor for intracerebral hemorrhage?	Hypertension
What are the miniature dilations that occur at bifurcations of small vessels in the brain secondary to hypertension?	Charcot-Bouchard aneurysms
What are the common places for Charcot-Bouchard aneurysms to occur?	Basal ganglion and thalamus
What type of intracranial hemorrhage presents as "the worst headache of my life?"	Subarachnoid hemorrhage
What are the common symptoms of a subarachnoid hemorrhage?	Vomiting, confusion, seizure
What is the most frequent cause of clinically significant subarachnoid hemorrhage?	Berry (or saccular) aneurysms
What are the most common sites of berry aneurysms?	Branch points of the circle of Willis
What are the most common vessels at which berry aneurysms develop?	ACoA PCoA MCA
A berry aneurysm in what area might present as bitemporal lower quadrantanopia and why?	ACoA—due to pressure on the superior optic chiasm
What is the term for yellow discoloration of cerebrospinal fluid (CSF) due to degraded red blood cells found in subarachnoid hemorrhage?	Xanthochromia
What is the most likely diagnosis in a patient presenting with "worst headache of my life" with a blown pupil and one eye deviating down and out?	Subarachnoid hemorrhage from a berry aneurysm in the PCoA compressing CN III

What are some of the medical diseases associated with an increased risk of berry aneurysms?

Adult polycystic kidney disease

Marfan syndrome

Ehlers-Danlos syndrome

What is the treatment of a leaking berry aneurysm?

Surgical clipping, ligation, or placement of an electrolytic platinum coil

Aside from intracranial bleeding, what is a major cause of morbidity and mortality associated with ruptured berry aneurysms?

Vasospasm

What is the term used to describe a neurologic event often involving transient aphasia that lasts less than 24 hours and resolves completely?

Transient ischemic attack (TIA)

What are TIAs usually a result of?

Carotid or vertebral emboli

TRAUMATIC BRAIN INJURY

What are the types of hemorrhages that can result from trauma to the head?

Epidural, subdural, subarachnoid, and parenchymal hemorrhages (Figs. 9.3, 9.4, and 9.5)

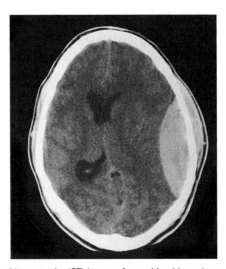

Figure 9.3 Computerized tomography (CT) image of an epidural hematoma. (*Courtesy of Michael Lipton, MD*)

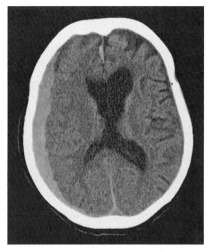

Figure 9.4 CT image of a subdural hematoma. (*Courtesy of Michael Lipton, MD*)

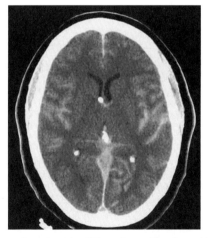

Figure 9.5 CT image of a subarachnoid hematoma. (*Courtesy of Michael Lipton, MD*)

What is the life-threatening complication of intracranial hemorrhage?

Herniation with subsequent brainstem compression

What effect does an intracranial hemorrhage have on cerebral perfusion pressure?

Decreased CPP due to increased intracranial pressure

What is the test of choice for diagnosing intracranial hemorrhage due to trauma?

CT scan without contrast

Name the intracranial hemorrhage associated with the following CT findings:

High attenuation (blood) present in the dark spaces normally filled with CSF	Subarachnoid
Biconvex "lentiform" hemorrhage	Epidural
Crescent-shaped hemorrhage that crosses suture lines	Subdural

Which type of hemorrhage is associated with skull fracture?

Epidural hematoma

What is the most common type of skull fracture that causes an epidural hematoma?

Temporal bone fracture

What is the source of blood in an epidural hematoma?

Middle meningeal artery

Between which two structures does the blood collect in an epidural hematoma?

1. Skull
2. Dura

Which type of hemorrhage might occur in a patient with blunt trauma to the head with loss of consciousness followed by a lucid interval and then rapid deterioration of mental status?

Epidural hematoma

Why is an epidural hematoma shaped like a biconvex lens?

Because the blood cannot cross suture lines.

Which type of intracranial hemorrhage is caused by venous blood?

Subdural hematoma

Between what two structures does the blood collect in a subdural hematoma?

1. Dura
2. Arachnoid

Which type of intracranial hemorrhage is more common in the elderly, alcoholics, and blunt trauma and may present hours to weeks after initial trauma?

Subdural hematoma

Why is the onset of symptoms often delayed in a subdural hematoma?

Bleeding is from the venous system (low pressure) and takes longer to accumulate and cause increased intracranial pressure (ICP).

What vessels tear to cause a subdural hematoma?	Bridging veins
What is a brain injury at the site of impact of trauma referred to as?	Coup injury
What is a brain injury on the opposite side of the brain from the site of impact referred to as?	Countrecoup injury
What are the four types of herniation syndromes that can occur after an intracranial hemorrhage?	1. Subfalcial herniation 2. Transtentorial (uncal) herniation 3. Cerebellar-foramen magnum herniation 4. Transcalvarial herniation
Describe each type of herniation:	Subfalcial: cingulate push under falx Uncal: uncus push through the tentorial incisure Cerebellar-foramen magnum herniation: cerebellum and medulla push through the foramen magnum Transcalvarial: brain pushes through fracture or surgical site
Which of the herniation syndromes presents with ipsilateral mydriasis and ptosis, contralateral homonymous hemianopsia, and ipsilateral paresis?	Transtentorial herniation
What accounts for the symptoms of uncal herniation?	Compression of the oculomotor nerve (CN III), optic tract, and contralateral cerebral peduncle
What is the treatment for epidural and subdural hematomas to prevent herniation of the brain?	Craniotomy with removal of the blood clot

HYDROCEPHALUS

What condition is characterized by an increase in CSF leading to an increase in ICP?	Hydrocephalus
What are the two classification of hydrocephalus?	1. Communicating hydrocephalus 2. Noncommunicating hydrocephalus

What is the classic finding on CT in hydrocephalus?	Dilated ventricles
In which spaces is CSF located?	Subarachnoid space and the ventricles
How much CSF is normally present in the subarachnoid space and ventricles?	Approximately 150 mL in adults
How much CSF is normally produced in one day?	Approximately 500 mL in adults
Which type of hydrocephalus has free flow of CSF between ventricles and subarachnoid space, and would show uniform dilation of ventricles on CT?	Communicating hydrocephalus
What are the three types of communicating hydrocephalus?	1. Hydrocephalus ex vacuo 2. Normal pressure hydrocephalus 3. Pseudotumor cerebri
What is the name of the condition characterized by ventricular dilation after substantial neuronal loss, such as in Alzheimer disease?	Hydrocephalus ex-vacuo
What is the name of the condition which classically presents with bladder incontinence, dementia, and ataxia?	Normal pressure hydrocephalus
What is an easy way to remember the triad of normal pressure hydrocephalus?	**W**et (incontinence) **W**acky (dementia) **W**obbly (ataxia)
What is the mechanism of normal pressure hydrocephalus?	Decreased resorption of CSF
Where is CSF resorbed?	Arachnoid villi within dural sinuses
What are some of the common etiologies of decreased resorption of CSF in normal pressure hydrocephalus?	About 50% idiopathic, subarachnoid hemorrhage, meningitis, trauma, and atherosclerosis
Why do patients with normal pressure hydrocephalus develop bladder incontinence?	Pressure on the subcortical fibers of the frontal lobe
What condition presents with headache and papilledema due to spontaneous increase in ICP without ventricular obstruction or mass, often without ventricular dilation on CT?	Pseudotumor cerebri

What is another name used to describe this condition?	Idiopathic intracranial hypertension
What is the common population in which pseudotumor cerebri occurs?	Young obese females
What is the mechanism behind the increased ICP?	Resistance to CSF outflow at the arachnoid villi
What treatments are usually effective in pseudotumor cerebri?	Acetazolamide and corticosteroids (both effectively decrease ICP)
What vascular lesion presents with symptoms similar to pseudotumor cerebri, including headache, ocular abnormalities, and idiopathic increase in ICP?	Venous sinus thrombosis
What are the common causes of venous sinus thrombosis?	Hypercoagulable state, extension of infection from paranasal sinuses, trauma, and pregnancy
What effect does increased ICP have on cerebral perfusion?	A severely elevated ICP can cause decreased perfusion.
What type of hydrocephalus has a blockage of CSF flow causing certain ventricles to be dilated on CT?	Noncommunicating hydrocephalus
What structures are blocked if the accumulation of CSF is in lateral, third, and fourth ventricles?	Foramina of Luschka/Magendie
What are the common etiologies of a blockage of the foramina of Luschka/Magendie?	Chronic meningitis Subarachnoid hemorrhage Atresia of foramina of Luschka/Magendie (congenital)
What structure is blocked if the lateral and third ventricles are dilated on CT?	Sylvian aqueduct
What is the etiology of a blockage of Sylvian aqueduct?	Congenital stenosis
What congenital malformation has a caudally displaced cerebellum and medulla through the foramen magnum, often causing a noncommunicating hydrocephalus?	Arnold-Chiari malformation

CLINICAL VIGNETTES

Make the diagnosis for the following patients:

A 50-year-old male with PMH of esophageal stricture and benign paroxysmal positional vertigo (BPPV) presents with headache and weakness in his right arm and leg. Patient fell on black ice a few hours ago, falling on the right side of his head with brief loss of consciousness (LOC). Physical examination: patient is confused with right pupil mydriatic and unresponsive to light, motor strength rated 3/5 in right bicep, triceps, quadriceps, and hamstrings. Visual field testing reveals intact central vision bilaterally with gross loss of peripheral vision on the right.

Uncal herniation with left posterior cerebral artery (PCA) occlusion and peripheral CN III compression

A 40-year-old male with history of polycystic kidney disease presents to the ER with the "worst headache of my life." Physical examination is significant for left eye deviating down and out. Laboratory tests reveal cerebrospinal fluid (CSF) is xanthochromic. CT demonstrates high attenuation in the CSF-filled spaces.

Subarachnoid hemorrhage from ruptured berry aneurysm

A 70-year-old male with history of carotid atherosclerosis and transient ischemic attacks (TIAs) presents with right-sided paralysis, sensory deficit, and aphasia. Physical examination is significant for right-sided weakness and sensory loss greater in upper extremity, right homonymous hemianopsia, and bruits heard over both carotids. Brain MRI confirms the suspected diagnosis.

Left (dominant) MCA cerebrovascular accident

An 18-year-old male presents with nausea, vomiting, headache, and "acting funny" 1 hour after being hit on the head by a stick. The patient had brief LOC but quickly recovered. CT shows a lens-shaped hyperdense mass on the right side adjacent to a fracture of the temporal bone.

Epidural hematoma

A 75-year-old male with history of alcoholism presents with headache, vomiting, and change in mental status. The patient's daughter states that he hit his head on a cabinet a few days ago but had no LOC at the time. CT shows a hyperdense crescent-shaped mass on the left side.

Subdural hematoma

A 70-year-old female with history of subarachnoid hemorrhage presents with trouble walking, increasing confusion, and loss of bladder control for 2 days. Physical examination is significant for ataxic gait, and failure of the mental status examination. CT shows extremely dilated ventricles.

Normal pressure hydrocephalus

CHAPTER 10

Intracranial Neoplasms

ADULT INTRACRANIAL TUMORS

What intracranial pathology has a higher mortality rate than intracranial neoplasms?	Stroke
In adults, what is the most common manifestation of a brain tumor?	Seizure
What other manifestations are seen in patients with intracranial tumors?	Altered mental function, headache, and dizziness
Are the majority of intracranial tumors in adults supratentorial or infratentorial?	Supratentorial
Name the five types of gliomas:	1. Glioblastoma multiforme (GBM) 2. Astrocytoma 3. Ependymoma 4. Medulloblastoma 5. Oligodendrocytoma
Which is the most common form of glioma?	Astrocytic tumors, including GBM (grade 4 astrocytoma)
What is a useful diagnostic marker in biopsy specimens of astrocytomas?	Glial fibrillary acidic protein (GFAP)
Where do astrocytomas (grades 1 and 2) in adults usually occur?	Cerebral hemispheres
What is the average survival period after the first symptom for astrocytomas?	5 to 6 years for cerebral astrocytomas 8+ years for cerebellar astrocytomas
Excision of which part of the cerebral astrocytoma can allow for survival in a functional state for many years?	Cystic cavity

What highly anaplastic astrocytoma is the most common primary brain tumor?

GBM

Describe the histopathologic features of GBM:

"Pseudopalisading" tumor cells border central areas of necrosis and hemorrhage.

What gross feature of GBM is the reason it is sometimes described as a "butterfly glioma"?

GBM tends to cross the corpus callosum.

What is the median survival for patients with GBM (grade 4) treated aggressively?

Approximately 12 months

What second most common primary brain tumor is associated with breast cancer and high estrogen states?

Meningioma

What is the characteristic histopathologic feature of this slow growing tumor?

Psammoma bodies and spindle cells arranged in concentrically arranged whorled pattern

What other tumors are associated with psammoma bodies?

Papillary adenocarcinoma of thyroid, serous cystadenocarcinoma of ovary, and mesothelioma

Which of these is the only benign tumor with psammoma bodies?

Meningioma

Which third most common primary brain tumor is characterized by Antoni A or B pattern of nuclei?

Schwannoma

What is the name used to describe a schwannoma localized to the eighth cranial nerve?

Acoustic neuroma

In which of the phakomatoses, or hereditary disease characterized by multiple hamartomas involving multiple tissues, are bilateral schwannomas found?

Neurofibromatosis type 2

What is the inheritance pattern of neurofibromatosis type 2?

Autosomal dominant, chromosome 22

From what structures do schwannomas, neurofibromas, and neurofibrosarcomas arise?

Cranial and peripheral nerves

What other tumor develops from myelin-producing cells?

Oligodendroglioma

Describe the typical growth pattern of an oligodendroglioma:

Benign, relatively slow-growing, usually originating in frontal lobes

Describe the characteristic histopathologic finding associated with oligodendroglioma:

"Fried egg cells" characterized by round nuclei with clear cytoplasm and often calcified

What intracranial tumor presents with symptoms of amenorrhea or galactorrhea in females, and diminished libido in males?

Prolactinoma (type of pituitary adenoma)

What visual field defect can result from a large prolactinoma and why?

Bitemporal hemianopsia—due to compression of the optic chiasm

What drugs are used in the pharmacologic treatment of prolactinomas?

Dopamine agonists: bromocriptine, pergolide, or cabergoline

Tumors of which three organs define multiple endocrine neoplasia type 1 (MEN 1) syndrome?

1. Pituitary
2. Parathyroid
3. Pancreas

What is the most common intraspinal adult tumor?

Myxopapillary ependymoma

What is the most frequent location for myxopapillary ependymoma?

Conus medullaris

Which tumor has assumed greater significance in the last two decades due to an increase in AIDS and immunosuppression?

Cerebral lymphoma

PEDIATRIC INTRACRANIAL TUMORS

What is the only type of childhood cancer that occurs with more frequency than intracranial neoplasms?

Leukemias

Where are the majority of pediatric intracranial tumors found?

Infratentorial

Based on anatomic location, children will more commonly present with what types of symptoms?

Cerebellar symptoms, such as unilateral ataxia and gait unsteadiness

Vomiting is a presenting symptom more often in tumors of which fossa?

Posterior cranial fossa

What is the most common pediatric intracranial tumor?

Pilocytic astrocytoma

Where do astrocytomas usually occur in children and adolescents?	Posterior fossa and optic nerves
Are pilocytic astrocytomas generally benign or malignant tumors?	Benign
What are the characteristic histopathologic findings of pilocytic astrocytoma?	Rosenthal fibers, bipolar cells, and microcysts
What highly malignant pediatric cerebellar tumor, found exclusively in the posterior fossa, is a type of primitive neuroectodermal tumor (PNET) that can compress the fourth ventricle causing hydrocephalus?	Medulloblastoma
Through what channels do medulloblastomas metastasize?	Cerebrospinal fluid (CSF) pathways
What are the characteristic histopathologic findings of medulloblastoma?	Rosettes or perivascular pseudorosette pattern of round blue cells that are highly radiosensitive
What other pediatric tumors are of neuroectodermal origin?	Neuroblastomas and retinoblastomas
What gene amplification is associated with neuroblastoma?	N-*myc* oncogene
What is the most common pediatric supratentorial tumor?	Craniopharyngioma
What is the embryologic origin of pituitary adenoma and craniopharyngioma?	Rathke's pouch
To what tumor of the jaw is craniopharyngioma histologically similar?	Ameloblastoma
What pediatric tumor arising from the ependymal cells lining the ventricle causes hydrocephalus and is characterized by blepharoplasts?	Ependymoma
What is the most common site of an ependymoma?	Fourth ventricle
What condition is associated with astrocytomas, cardiac rhabdomyomas, and facial angiofibromas, can present as seizures, and has an inheritance pattern with incomplete penetrance?	Tuberous sclerosis

Which type of astrocytoma is pathognomonic for tuberous sclerosis?	Subependymal giant cell astrocytomas
What are the main physical findings of tuberous sclerosis?	Flesh-colored papules on the face (adenoma sebaceum) and in the nail beds (ungula fibromas), and flesh-colored patches on the trunk (shagreen patches)
Name two diseases in which hamartomas and neoplasms can both be found.	1. Tuberous sclerosis 2. Neurofibromatosis type 1
What are the classic findings of neurofibromatosis type 1 (von Recklinghausen disease)?	Café-au-lait spots, neurofibromas, multiple freckles, optic gliomas, and iris hamartomas (Lisch nodules)
What is the inheritance pattern of neurofibromatosis type 1?	Autosomal dominant, chromosome 17

MISCELLANEOUS

What syndrome causing defect of the $p53$ tumor suppressor gene is associated with brain tumors?	Li-Fraumeni syndrome
What other types of tumors can result from Li-Fraumeni syndrome?	Breast cancer, leukemia, and sarcomas
What highly vascular tumor of the cerebellum is characterized by foamy cells that produce erythropoietin, and can cause secondary polycythemia?	Hemangioblastoma
Hemangioblastoma is associated with what syndrome when found with retinoblastoma?	von Hippel-Lindau (VHL) syndrome
What is the inheritance pattern of VHL syndrome?	Autosomal dominant, chromosome 3
What other findings are common in VHL syndrome?	Retinal hemangioblastomas, pheochromocytomas, and cysts in the kidney and pancreas
Retinoblastoma increases one's risk for what type of cancer?	Osteosarcoma
What features do teratomas, germinomas, choriocarcinomas, and endodermal sinus carcinomas have in common?	They can all occur as intracranial midline germline tumors.

SEQUELAE AND TREATMENT

What are the three most common herniations due to a mass effect?

1. Subfalcial herniation
2. Uncal herniation
3. Cerebellar-foramen magnum herniation

What is a false localizing sign?

A focal neurologic sign caused by mass effect from a lesion elsewhere

Which one of the three herniations most commonly produces a false localizing sign?

Uncal herniation (transtentorial)

Which cranial nerve does an uncal herniation most commonly involve and with which manifestation?

Ipsilateral oculomotor (CN III) causing dilation of the ipsilateral pupil with ptosis

What potentially fatal hemorrhages are produced when the midbrain is crushed between a herniating temporal lobe and the opposite leaf of tentorium?

Duret hemorrhages

What ultimately is the cause of death from intracranial tumors?

Cerebral edema and increased intracranial pressure (ICP)

What type of sequelae result from proteases released by tumor cells?

Vasogenic edema by weakening the blood-brain barrier and allowing passage of serum protein

Is gray or white matter more vulnerable to effects of vasogenic edema and why?

White matter, possibly due to its looser structural organization offering less resistance to fluid under pressure

Which kind of edema results mainly from hypoxic ischemic injury?

Cytotoxic or cellular edema

How is brain edema and increased ICP from vasogenic edema generally treated therapeutically prior to treatment of the underlying disease?

High potency glucocorticoids (dexamethasone), thought to reduce permeability of endothelium

Which is the most common osmotic solute used to decrease edema?

Mannitol

What is the mechanism of the transient effectiveness of hyperventilation to reduce edema?

Resulting respiratory alkalosis causes a vasoconstriction and decreased cerebral blood flow.

CLINICAL VIGNETTES

Make the diagnosis for the following patients:

A 6-year-old male with a 4-month history of repeated vomiting, listlessness, and morning headaches now presents with stumbling gait and positional dizziness. He was sent home by the primary doctor (PMD) with an initial diagnosis of gastrointestinal (GI) disease or abdominal migraine 3 months ago. Physical examination is significant for papilledema; diplopia caused by lateral strabismus, nystagmus, and positive Romberg sign. Head tilt to the right side is present. MRI shows high signal intensity on both T1- and T2-weighted images—left-sided heterogenous enhancement adjacent to and fungating into the fourth ventricle. Pathology shows small cells closely packed with hyperchromatic nuclei, little cytoplasm, many mitoses, and pseudorosette pattern.

Medulloblastoma

A 61-year-old woman with history of neurofibromatosis type 2 presents with headache, slowly progressive spastic weakness and numbness of the left leg, incontinence, and worsening mental status. Neurologic signs, including focal seizures, have been present for many years. There is a family history of breast cancer. Physical examination is significant for papilledema. CT scan with contrast shows dural-based enhancing right-sided softball-sized tumor. Pathology shows psammoma bodies.

Meningioma

A 30-year-old male with history of AIDS presents with behavioral and personality changes, confusion, dizziness, focal cerebral signs, and family history of Wiskott-Aldrich and ataxia telangiectasia. CT scan shows dense, homogenous enhancing periventricular mass. Pathology confirms presence of Epstein-Barr virus (EBV) in lesion.

Primary cerebral lymphoma

A 58-year-old with history of lung cancer and multiple myeloma presents with headache, seizures, vomiting, behavioral abnormalities, ataxia, aphasia, and focal weakness progressively worsening over the past few months with 17% body weight loss. Bone scan reveals lytic lesions and CT scan shows multiple nodular deposits of tumor in the brain. MRI rules out brain abscesses.

Metastatic carcinoma

A 4-year-old male presents with retarded height velocity and decreased weight gain, vomiting, difficulty in swallowing, vague abdominal pain, vertigo, and head tilting over the past 14 months. Physical examination is significant for papilledema, vertical downbeating nystagmus, and paresthesia of toes bilaterally. CT scan shows mass growing into the fourth ventricle and signs of perivascular rosettes. Pathology shows presence of blepharoplasts (basal ciliary bodies near nucleus).

Ependymoma

A 58-year-old male with a 2-month history of headache and left intraorbital pain now has seizures. Physical examination is significant for papilledema. MRI shows a 2 × 2.5 × 1.5 cm irregular variegated lesion on the left temporal lobe extending through the corpus callosum to the right hemisphere. The T1-weighted image of the lesion demonstrates low intensity, but T2 demonstrates higher intensity with implication of cerebral necrosis, and vasogenic edema. There is homogeneous enhancement of the lesion after gadolinium injection. Pathology reveals foci of necrosis with pseudopalisading of malignant nuclei and endothelial cell proliferation, leading to a "glomeruloid" structure.

Glioblastoma multiforme

A 50-year-old with a 7-month history of high-pitched tinnitus, like that of a steam kettle, and facial pain presents with use of unaccustomed ear in telephone conversations coinciding with attacks of vertigo and gait abnormalities. Family history is notable for von Recklinghausen disease. Physical examination is significant for sensory deficits localizing to all branches of trigeminal and facial nerves. CSF protein is markedly elevated. Contrast-enhanced CT reveals 2.5-cm mass projecting into cerebellopontine angle.

Schwannoma

A 6-year-old child with a 7-week history of complaints of it "always being dark," urination of 10 to 12 times per day, drinking multiple liters of fluid a day now presents with headache and vomiting. The child has signs of delayed physical and mental development. Physical examination is significant for bitemporal hemianopia and papilledema. MRI reveals increased signal on T1-weighted image. CT shows calcium deposits in suprasellar region. Pathology demonstrates dark albuminous fluid, cholesterol crystals, and calcium deposits in cyst.

Craniopharyngioma

A 35-year-old male with a 3-year history of seizures presents with weakness of the right leg. Physical examination is significant for papilledema. CT demonstrates hypodense calcified mass near the left cortical surface with well-defined borders. Pathology reveals sheets of regular cells with spherical nuclei containing finely granular chromatin surrounded by a clear halo of cytoplasm, "fried egg cells."

Oligodendroglioma

A 12-year-old presents with headache, vomiting, and gait unsteadiness. Physical examination is significant for unilateral ataxia and positive Romberg sign. MRI T1-weighted image shows isointense sharply demarcated mass with smooth borders and little associated edema. T2-weighted image shows hyperintensity and marked enhancement after gadolinium injection. Pathology demonstrates increased staining of biopsy with glial fibrillary acidic protein (GFAP).

Pilocytic astrocytoma

A 22-year-old athlete with a 3-month history of dizziness and decreasing exercise tolerance with occasional chest pain presents with complaint of falling over to the left side. Family history is notable for von Hippel-Lindau disease. Physical examination is significant for retinal angioma. Lab studies reveal slight LFT (liver function test) derangements and increased amylase and lipase. MRI shows mass with associated edema in left cerebellar hemisphere, as well as hepatic and pancreatic cysts. Vertebral angiogram defines a hypervascular nodule with dilated draining veins.

Hemangioblastoma

A 36-year-old female with a 4-month history of headache and loss of menstruation realized after cessation of birth control pills presents with complaint of staining her bra. She has also been involved in multiple motor vehicle accidents in the last few months while changing lanes. Menarche occurred at age 12. Physical examination is significant for papilledema and galactorrhea. Lab studies reveal serum prolactin level is 220 ng/mL. Coronal MRI shows nonenhancing nodule inferior to the optic chiasm. Administration of bromocriptine resulted in normalization of prolactin levels, regression of mass, reinitiation of menstrual flow, and disappearance of visual field scotomas.

Pituitary adenoma (prolactinoma)

A 9-year-old male with no significant PMH is brought in by his parents for concern of multiple freckles in the axilla and groin despite continual sunscreen use and hyperpigmented patches of skin on his abdomen and arms. Polymerase chain reaction (PCR) studies found a mutation localized to chromosome 17. Further evaluation revealed brown spots on the irises bilaterally.

Neurofibromatosis type 1

CHAPTER 11

Infectious Diseases

MENINGITIS

What are common symptoms of meningitis?	Headache, fever, vomiting, photophobia, and stiff neck (nuchal rigidity)
In what age group is nuchal rigidity typically not seen?	Children <1 year and patients with altered mental status
What other age group does not present with classic symptoms?	Elderly

Name the appropriate signs associated with meningitis:

Inability to touch one's chin to chest	Meningismus
Patient lies supine with legs flexed to 90° and examiner cannot extend the knee	Kernig sign
Patient lies supine and flexion of the neck results in involuntary flexion of the knees	Brudzinski sign

Name the type of meningitis associated with the following cerebrospinal fluid (CSF) findings:

Numerous polymorphonuclear cells (PMN/neutrophils), decreased glucose (less than two-thirds of the serum glucose concentration), and increased protein	Bacterial meningitis
Increased lymphocytes, moderately increased protein, and normal CSF pressure	Viral meningitis
Increased lymphocytes, moderately elevated protein, and elevated CSF pressure	Fungal meningitis

Name the appropriate organism(s) associated with following clinical and pathologic features:

Most common cause of bacterial meningitis in adults	*Streptococcus pneumoniae* (50%)
Second most common cause of bacterial meningitis in adults	*Neisseria meningitidis* (25%)
Most common cause of bacterial meningitis in neonates	*Streptococcus agalactiae* (group B Strep, [GBS])
Other causes of meningitis in neonates	*Escherichia coli, Listeria monocytogenes*
Increased risk with splenectomy or impaired humoral immunity	*S. pneumoniae, Haemophilus influenza, N. meningitidis*
Associated with petechial rash on trunk and extremities	*N. meningitidis*
Associated with Waterhouse-Friderichsen syndrome (hemorrhagic destruction of adrenal cortex)	*N. meningitidis*
Increased risk with premature rupture of membranes, chorioamnionitis in mother	GBS
Associated with transplacental transmission	GBS, *E. coli, L. monocytogenes*
Introduction of vaccine has dramatically reduced the incidence of infection in the last 10 to 15 years	*H. influenza*

Name the appropriate treatment for the following types of meningitis:

Pneumococcal meningitis	Ceftriaxone + vancomycin
Meningococcal meningitis	Penicillin G
Close contacts of a patient with meningococcal meningitis	Rifampin prophylaxis
GBS meningitis	Ampicillin

Name the appropriate organism(s) associated with the following clinical and pathologic features:

Most common cause of viral meningitis	Echovirus
Other organisms that cause viral meningitis	Coxsackie virus, adenovirus, herpes simplex virus (HSV), HIV, cytomegalovirus (CMV), and Epstein-Barr virus (EBV)
Four causes of fungal meningitis	1. *Cryptococcus* 2. *Coccidioides* 3. *Aspergillus* 4. Histoplasmosis
India ink stain used to detect organism in CSF	*Cryptococcus*
Basilar enhancement on MRI	*Mycobacterium tuberculosis* (TB meningitis)
Amebic meningitis associated with swimming in lakes	*Naegleria fowleri*

What symptoms are seen in TB meningitis?	Weight loss and night sweats
What is the prognosis of amebic meningitis from *N. fowleri*?	95% mortality within 1 week

Name the appropriate treatment for the following:

Viral meningitis	Symptomatic support for fever and pain
Fungal meningitis	Amphotericin B followed by fluconazole
TB meningitis	Isoniazid (INH) rifampin + pyrazinamide + ethambutol

What vitamin supplement should be given with INH?	Pyridoxine (B_6)

List the complications of meningitis:	Cerebral edema
	Seizures
	Syndrome of inappropriate antidiuretic hormone (SIADH)
	Subdural effusion
	Deafness
	Hydrocephalus

ENCEPHALITIS

To what encephalitic infections are babies susceptible?	TORCH infections: Toxoplasmosis, Other (syphilis), Rubella, CMV, and HSV
When is the worst time for mothers to be infected with a TORCH disease and why?	The first trimester—organogenesis occurs in weeks 3 to 8
During which trimesters is a fetus most susceptible to congenital syphilis?	Second and third trimesters

Name the organism(s) associated with the following clinical and pathologic features:

Spreads from cats to humans and causes periventricular calcifications with congenital infection	Toxoplasmosis
Congenital infection associated with cataracts, chorioretinitis, patent ductus arteriosus, and "blueberry muffin baby"	Rubella
Congenital infection associated with diffuse intracranial calcifications	CMV
Congenital infection associated with vesicular skin lesions and conjunctivitis	HSV
Congenital infection associated with blood-tinged nasal secretions (snuffles), osteochondritis, Hutchinson teeth (notching of permanent upper two incisors), saddle nose, and hearing loss	*Treponema pallidum* (syphilis)
Babies born with focal cerebral calcification, microcephaly, and chorioretinitis should be tested for which infections?	Toxoplasmosis and CMV
Which TORCH infections are the most common causes of congenital hydrocephalus?	Toxoplasmosis and CMV
What are the common neurologic findings in congenital syphilis?	Basilar meningitis, cranial neuropathies (CN II, III, VII, VIII), congenital blindness, hydrocephalus, and infarction from vasculitis (endarteritis)
What is the pathophysiology of blueberry muffin skin?	Thrombocytopenia causes purple purpura and petechiae

Name the organism(s) associated with the following clinical and pathologic features:

The most common cause of a space-occupying lesion in AIDS patients and appears radiographically as multiple ring-enhancing mass lesions	Toxoplasmosis (primary cerebral lymphoma is the second most common cause of a space-occupying lesion in AIDS patients)
Most common cause of viral encephalitis, most frequently affecting teenagers and young adults	HSV
Associated with findings of RBCs in the CSF and particularly affects the temporal lobe	HSV
Other causes of viral encephalitis	Arboviruses, CMV, rabies, and HIV
Transmitted by mosquitoes and ticks and includes St. Louis encephalitis virus, Eastern equine encephalitis virus, and Western equine encephalitis virus	Arboviruses
Acquired through bites of dogs, raccoons, and skunks and associated with hydrophobia	Rabies
Histologic findings of neuronal degeneration and Negri bodies in hippocampus and cerebellum (eosinophilic intracytoplasmic inclusions)	Rabies
Histologic findings of giant cells with eosinophilic inclusions in both the nucleus and cytoplasm	CMV

Name the appropriate treatment for the following encephalitides:

Toxoplasmosis encephalitis	Bactrim (trimethoprim/sulfamethoxazole)
Herpes encephalitis	Acyclovir
Rabies encephalitis	Active and passive immunizations given prior to the onset of clinical manifestations
CMV encephalitis	Ganciclovir

What cells are responsible for viral entry into the nervous system in HIV infection?	Monocytes are a reservoir for the virus and penetrate the blood-brain barrier.

What is the clinical manifestation of HIV on the nervous system?	Progressive dementia, also known as AIDS-related dementia complex
What virus is associated with subacute sclerosing panencephalitis (SSPE), a slowly progressive and usually fatal disease?	Rubeola virus (measles)

NEUROSYPHILIS

Which stages of syphilis are associated with central nervous system (CNS) damage?	Secondary and tertiary syphilis
What are the serologic tests available for detection of syphilis?	VDRL Rapid plasma reagent (RPR) Fluorescent treponemal antigen absorption (FTA-ABS) Microhemagglutination assay for *T. pallidum* (MHA-TP)
A false-positive in which of these tests is associated with systemic lupus erythematosus?	VDRL
T. pallidum can be seen under what kind of microscopy?	Darkfield microscopy
What CNS manifestation is associated with secondary syphilis?	Syphilitic meningitis
What are the features of syphilitic meningitis?	Headache, stiff neck, fever, and CSF containing high lymphocytes, high protein, and low glucose
What are the other two CNS manifestations of syphilis?	1. Meningovascular syphilis 2. Parenchymatous syphilis
What are the consequences of meningovascular syphilis?	Vascular insufficiency or stroke due to endarteritis
What are some of the symptoms of parenchymatous syphilis?	Dementia, tremor, and dysarthria
What clinical findings are associated with parenchymatous syphilis?	Tabes dorsalis and Argyll Robertson pupils
Name the condition associated with tertiary syphilis that is characterized by degeneration of dorsal columns resulting in impaired proprioception and ataxia:	Tabes dorsalis

What is the name of the condition associated with tertiary syphilis where the pupils accommodate but do not react to light (prostitute's pupils)?

Argyll Robertson pupils

MISCELLANEOUS

What are some risk factors for cerebral abscess?

Trauma (penetrating skull injuries), spread of infections from other sites including middle ear, paranasal sinuses, and infective endocarditis

What is the most common risk factor for cerebral abscess?

Middle ear infection

What are complications of cerebral abscesses?

Increased intracranial pressure and rupture into the ventricles—fatal unless treated

Which parasitic disease is characterized by cyst formation that eventually results in an intense inflammatory reaction and encephalitis and is endemic to Latin America?

Neurocysticercosis

What organism is responsible for neurocysticercosis?

Larval stage of *Taenia solium* (pork tapeworm)

Which viral illness transmitted by fecal-oral route results in destruction of anterior horn cells, and presents with symptoms of hyporeflexia, muscle weakness, and atrophy?

Poliomyelitis

Which organism is responsible for poliomyelitis?

Poliovirus

What are the infectious agents resistant to heating and other sterilization techniques responsible for Creutzfeldt-Jakob disease (CJD)?

Prions

What are the clinical features of CJD?

Progressive ataxia, dementia, and tremor

What change in the prion protein (PrP) is responsible for the etiology of CJD?

Conversion from predominantly alpha-helix (PrPc) to beta-pleated sheet (PrPsc)

| What are the characteristic histopathologic findings of CJD? | Spongiform encephalopathy characterized by neuronal vacuolization and cysts in gray matter without an associated inflammatory reaction |

CLINICAL VIGNETTES

Make the diagnosis for the following patients:

A 45-year-old female presents with fever, neck stiffness, and photophobia. Physical examination is significant for positive Kernig and Brudzinski signs. Labs show elevated protein and decreased glucose in CSF with gram-positive diplococci.

Meningitis: *S. pneumoniae*

A 3-year-old male presents with fever, irritability, vomiting, and petechial skin rash. Labs show elevated protein and decreased glucose in CSF with gram-negative diplococci.

Meningitis: *N. meningitides*

A 42-year-old HIV positive male presents with chronic low-grade fever and chronic headache and neck stiffness. CSF findings include India ink staining of yeast with a halo.

Cryptococcal meningitis

A 50-year-old recent immigrant from Mexico presents with severe headache, vomiting, papilledema, and altered mental status. History is significant for potential consumption of undercooked pork. CT shows calcified intracranial cysts.

Neurocysticercosis

A 60-year-old male with previous history of syphilis presents with ataxia. Physical examination shows loss of vibration and joint position sense in lower extremities and loss of pupillary light reflex, but normal accommodation reflex.

Tertiary syphilis

A 53-year-old HIV positive female presents with headache, altered mental status, and seizures. She has two pet cats. CT shows multiple ring-enhancing lesions.

Toxoplasmosis

A 4-year-old boy with past history of persistent bloody nasal discharge, presents with progressive hearing loss, notched incisors, and flattened nose.

Congenital syphilis

A 3-week-old girl presents with bilateral cataracts and a continuous machinery murmur best heard over the left pulmonary area. Mother reports that she had a diffuse rash and fever during her first trimester.

Congenital rubella

CHAPTER 12

Demyelinating Diseases

How does demyelination change the following properties of an axon?

Capacitance	↑
Membrane resistance	↓
Conduction velocity	↓
Length constant	↓
Time constant	↑

CAUSES OF DEMYELINATION

Name the inflammatory demyelinating diseases:

Multiple sclerosis (MS)

Progressive multifocal leukoencephalopathy (PML)

Acute disseminated encephalomyelitis (ADEM)

Guillain-Barré syndrome

Name the hereditary demyelinating diseases:

Krabbe disease

Metachromatic leukodystrophy

Adrenoleukodystrophy

Charcot-Marie-Tooth (CMT) disease

Pelizaeus-Merzbacher disease

Canavan disease

INFLAMMATORY DEMYELINATING DISEASE

What are the clinical manifestations of PML?

Mental deterioration, vision loss, speech disturbances, ataxia, and paralysis

What cell type does JC virus, the etiologic agent in PML, preferentially infect?

Oligodendrocytes

What patients get PML?

Immunocompromised

Which inflammatory demyelinating disease can follow vaccination or viral infection (most commonly measles)?

ADEM

Where is the demyelination and inflammation located in ADEM?

Perivenular area

List some viruses that can cause ADEM:

Measles (most common cause)

Mumps

Rubella

Epstein-Barr virus

Influenza

Parainfluenza

What bacterial infections can also cause ADEM?

Mycoplasma

Borrelia burgdorferi

Leptospira

β-hemolytic streptococci

Autoimmune response to what protein has been associated with ADEM?

Myelin basic protein (MBP)

What often-fatal form of ADEM is characterized by necrotizing venular vasculitis?

Acute hemorrhagic encephalomyelitis (AHEM)

Which disease manifests as self-limiting ascending paralysis associated with prior infection or vaccination?

Guillain-Barré syndrome

Infection with what bacteria is associated with roughly 25% cases of Guillain-Barré syndrome?

Campylobacter jejuni

Infection with what other pathogens has been associated with Guillain-Barré syndrome?

HIV, cytomegalovirus (CMV), Epstein-Barr virus, and *Mycoplasma pneumoniae*

What are the histopathologic findings in Guillain-Barre syndrome?	Perivascular lymphocytes, perivenous demyelination
What is the immunopathogenesis of Guillain-Barré syndrome?	Molecular mimicry
What is molecular mimicry?	An immune response to foreign antigens that resemble self-antigens
Which self-antigen is the immune response directed against in Guillain-Barré syndrome?	Gangliosides located at the nodes of Ranvier
What cerebrospinal fluid (CSF) abnormalities are associated with Guillain-Barré syndrome?	Increased CSF protein without an increase in cells (albuminocytologic dissociation)
What is the biggest risk for mortality in Guillain-Barré syndrome?	Respiratory muscle paralysis (requires mechanical ventilation)
What is the treatment for Guillain-Barré syndrome?	Plasmapheresis or IV immunoglobulin (equally effective)
What is the incidence of MS?	1/1000
What is the typical age of onset for MS?	Between 20 and 40 years of age
Are there gender differences in incidence of MS?	Female to male ratio = 2:1
What human leukocyte antigen (HLA) type is associated with MS?	HLA-DR2
What geographic factor has been associated with MS?	Incidence correlated with ↑ distance from equator during first 15 years of life
What socioeconomic factors have been associated with increased risk of MS?	High socioeconomic status
Autoimmune T-cell response to which protein has been implicated in MS?	MBP
Autoantibodies directed against which protein have been found in patients with MS?	Myelin oligodendrocyte glycoprotein (MOG)
What is it called when protein electrophoresis of the CSF shows two to five bands of immunoglobulins?	Oligoclonal banding

What CSF abnormalities are associated with MS?	Increased mononuclear cells and oligoclonal banding (indicates intrathecal IgG production)
Besides MS, what other diseases can be associated with CSF oligoclonal banding?	Systemic lupus erythematosus (SLE) Neurosarcoidosis Subacute sclerosing panencephalitis (SSPE) Subarachnoid hemorrhage Syphilis Central nervous system (CNS) lymphoma
What immune cells are found in acute MS plaques?	T cells and macrophages are found around venules (perivenular cuffing) and extend into adjacent white matter
What cells scavenge the myelin debris in an MS plaque?	Macrophages and microglial cells
What cell type proliferates as the acute MS plaque evolves to a more chronic plaque, causing gliosis?	Astrocytes
Name the chronic plaque characterized by gliosis and partial remyelination:	Shadow plaque
What cytokines play an important role in pathogenesis of MS?	Interleukin (IL)-2, tumor necrosis factor (TNF)-α, and interferon (IFN)-γ
What are some of the early findings in MS patients?	Weakness as well as visual and sensory disturbances
What symptoms of MS constitute what is known as Charcot triad?	Nystagmus, intention tremor, and scanning speech
What is the other well-known Charcot triad associated with cholangitis?	Jaundice, fever, and upper quadrant pain
Demyelination in what neural structure can account for all three symptoms of Charcot triad?	Cerebellum
Name the common cause of diplopia and nystagmus in MS patients resulting from lesion of the medial longitudinal fasciculus (MLF):	Internuclear ophthalmoplegia

Describe the deficits that result from internuclear ophthalmoplegia due to demyelination of the right MLF:

When looking to the left, the right eye does not adduct and the left eye displays nystagmus.

What lesion accounts for decreased visual acuity and color desaturation in an MS patient?

Optic neuritis

What is Lhermitte phenomenon?

Flexion of the neck causes electrical sensation down the neck and shoulders, associated with MS

Name the four different clinical courses of MS that have been described:

1. Relapsing-remitting
2. Primary-progressive
3. Secondary-progressive
4. Progressive-relapsing

How common is the relapsing-remitting course?

Most common course (~85% of cases)

What proportion of these patients develop secondary progression?

Approximately half

Name the clinical course of MS associated with the following description:

Attacks with acute neurologic signs, followed by recovery

Relapsing-remitting

Slow but nearly continuous worsening of the disease without distinct attacks or remissions

Primary-progressive

Initially relapsing-remitting, followed by steadily worsening course

Secondary-progressive

Steadily worsening disease with clear acute attacks, and intervening periods defined by continuing progression

Progressive-relapsing

How does pregnancy affect flare-ups of MS?

Patients have fewer attacks during pregnancy, but more in the first 3 months postpartum, making the absolute number of attacks equal to that of a nonpregnant individual.

How are acute attacks of MS treated?

Glucocorticoid treatment

What immunomodulator medications are used in daily management of MS?

IFN-1a (Avonex), IFN-β1a (Rebif), IFN-β1b (Betaseron), glatiramer acetate (Copaxone)

List some poor prognostic factors for MS:	High relapse rate, short interval between first and second attack, older age of onset, early cerebellar involvement
What new MS drug is associated with a risk of PML?	Natalizumab (Tysabri)
What is the mechanism of action of natalizumab?	Anti-integrin-4 antibody suppresses leukocyte migration.
For what other autoimmune disease has natalizumab been given FDA approval?	Crohn disease

HEREDITARY DEMYELINATING DISEASES

Name the leukodystrophy associated with the following:

Caused by an autosomal recessive deficiency in beta-galactocerebrosidase	Krabbe disease
Caused by an autosomal recessive deficiency in arylsulfatase A	Metachromatic leukodystrophy
Caused by an X-linked inability to process long chain fatty acids	Adrenoleukodystrophy
Galactosphingosine builds up in oligodendrocytes, causing their destruction	Krabbe disease
Progressive spastic paraparesis in teenage boys with a history of adrenal insufficiency during childhood	Adrenoleukodystrophy
Globoid bodies (multinucleated macrophage aggregates)	Krabbe disease
What is the inheritance pattern in CMT disease?	Most commonly autosomal dominant, but can also be autosomal recessive, X-linked, or sporadic
What is damaged in CMT disease?	CMT disease is a hereditary peripheral neuropathy of both motor and sensory nerves. CMT type 1 is characterized by demyelination and type 2 by axonal degeneration.
What happens to conduction velocity in CMT disease?	Conduction velocity decreases in both motor and sensory nerves in type I disease (normal in type II).

What are the findings on nerve biopsy in CMT disease?	Onion bulbs characteristic of hypertrophic demyelinating neuropathy
What are common clinical findings in CMT disease?	Muscle weakness and atrophy beginning distally and progressing proximally, impaired sensation, and areflexia
What is age of onset for CMT disease?	First to second decade
What is the X-linked disease of defective myelination due to mutation in the proteolipid protein gene?	Pelizaeus-Merzbacher disease

CLINICAL VIGNETTES

Make the diagnosis for the following patients:

A 29-year-old woman from Boston complains of recent transient blindness and double vision. On physical examination, she has intention tremor, nystagmus, and scanning speech. On neck flexion, she reports a painful sensation in her neck and shoulder. MRI reveals scattered white matter plaques. CSF studies demonstrate oligoclonal banding.

Multiple sclerosis

A 60-year-old female complains of foot drop and recent onset of muscle weakness in her legs. She reports that numbness and tingling in her legs began 2 weeks after an upper respiratory infection. She is also beginning to notice weakness in hands and arms. Physical examination demonstrates weakness in the extremities and increased protein in CSF without cells.

Guillain-Barré syndrome

A 15-year-old male complains of progressive weakness in his lower leg. He reports that one of his older siblings had a similar problem. Physical examination reveals atrophy of the calf muscles, high foot arches, and palpable thickening of nerves.

Charcot-Marie-Tooth disease

CHAPTER 13

Seizures

What is a seizure?	Abnormal excessive and synchronous firing of neurons resulting in alterations in movement, sensation, or consciousness
What is epilepsy?	Chronic condition characterized by recurrent seizures
What is the most common etiology of epilepsy?	Idiopathic
What is the prevalence of epilepsy in the United States?	About 1%
In which age groups is the incidence of seizures highest?	Infancy and elderly
What is the most likely etiology of seizures in elderly patients?	Primary or metastatic brain tumors
What is the typical cause of seizures in infants?	Fever (Febrile seizures)

PARTIAL SEIZURES

What is meant by the term partial seizure?	Partial seizures originate in a focus and do not involve both hemispheres
What are the two classes of partial seizures?	1. Simple 2. Complex
What is the major difference between simple and complex partial seizures?	Consciousness is altered in complex partial seizures, but not in simple partial seizures.
What is the term used to describe hallucinations that precede complex partial seizures?	Auras

What types of auras precede the onset and progression of complex partial seizures?

Sensory (usually visual or auditory)

Déjà vu (already seen) or jamais vu (never seen)

Sudden emotions (particularly fear or anxiety)

Complex partial seizures most commonly have a focus in which region of the brain?

Medial temporal lobe

What are the major risk factors associated with adult onset of complex partial seizures, as often seen in temporal lobe epilepsy?

Febrile seizure in infancy and bacterial meningitis

What is the characteristic finding on brain imaging in cases of temporal lobe epilepsy?

Medial temporal sclerosis

Laughter is the automatism of which unusual kind of seizure associated with hypothalamic hamartomas and precocious puberty?

Gelastic seizure

What are the four types of simple partial seizures?

1. Motor
2. Sensory
3. Autonomic
4. Psychic

What determines the type of simple partial seizure?

Location of the focus

Where is the typical focus of a simple motor seizure?

Frontal lobe (especially motor or premotor areas)

Visual manifestations such as light flashes and unformed images suggest seizure activity in which cortical region?

Occipital

Sensations of vertigo as a manifestation of sensory seizure indicate activity in which cortical area?

Superior temporal

Gustatory hallucinations are indicative of aberrant activity in which cortical area?

Insula

The generally unpleasant odors, such as burning rubber, associated with olfactory auras indicate seizure activity in which region of the cortex?

Inferior temporal or uncus

What are some of the manifestations of a psychic seizure?	Difficulty thinking, sudden emotions, and feelings of déjà vu (already seen) or jamais vu (never seen)
What type of cortical area is involved in psychic seizures?	Association cortices that integrate across multiple modalities

GENERALIZED SEIZURES

What is the term used to describe a seizure that is initiated in both hemispheres of the cerebral cortex?	Primary generalized
What is the term used to describe a seizure that starts focally and spreads to involve both hemispheres of the cerebral cortex?	Secondary generalized
What are the different types of generalized seizures?	Absence Myoclonic Atonic Tonic Tonic-clonic
What is an older term used to describe tonic-clonic seizures?	Grand mal
Which type of primary generalized seizure, often manifest as staring spells, can be mistaken as daydreaming?	Absence seizure
What is an older term used to describe absence seizures?	Petit mal
In what age group are absence seizures typically seen?	Children (ages 5–15)
What type of neuron is believed to be the source of aberrant activity in absence seizures?	Thalamic relay neurons
What ion channel is targeted by drugs used to treat absence seizures?	Calcium T-channel
Agonists of which receptor on thalamic relay neurons can exacerbate absence seizures?	$GABA_B$ receptors

What technique can be used clinically to provoke absence seizures?	Hyperventilation
What motor manifestations are sometimes seen with absence seizures?	Blinking, eye rolling, lip smacking, chewing, and fumbling of fingers
What is the characteristic EEG finding in children with absence seizures?	3-Hz spike and wave
What is the drug of choice for simple absence seizures?	Ethosuximide
Which type of primary generalized seizure involves repetitive muscle contractions?	Myoclonic
What epilepsy syndrome, seen in young adults, is sometimes brought on by fatigue or alcohol ingestion?	Juvenile myoclonic epilepsy
What drug, sometimes used to treat absence seizures, is used as the first-line agent in treatment of myoclonic epilepsies?	Valproate
What type of primary generalized seizure, also known as a "drop attack" involves sudden loss of muscle tones?	Atonic seizures
Which type of primary generalized seizure, often occurring during sleep, manifests as sudden increases in muscle tone?	Tonic seizures
During what type of generalized seizure would you find a patient apneic (not breathing) with dilated and unreactive pupils?	Tonic-clonic
How much do patients usually recall in the postictal (after seizure) period?	Nothing—patients are usually confused and amnesic.
What is the term used to describe a generalized seizure lasting >30 minutes, or multiple seizures without a lucid interictal conscious period?	*Status epilepticus*
What is the mortality rate of status epilepticus?	20%–30%
What are the common complications of status epilepticus?	Hyperthermia, acidosis, and myoglobinuria

What is the proper treatment for status epilepticus?	Benzodiazepines (diazepam or lorazepam)
	Fosphenytoin
Why are parenteral diazepam, lorazepam, and fosphenytoin preferred in the treatment of status epilepticus?	Rapid onset
	Titratable dose

PEDIATRIC EPILEPSY SYNDROMES

Name the epilepsy syndrome described below:

Manifest as nocturnal twitching, numbness, or tingling in the face or tongue	Benign Rolandic (aka benign childhood epilepsy)
Onset in early childhood, usually consists of drop attacks from tonic or atonic seizures, which are difficult to control, and generally involves substantial intellectual impairment	Lennox-Gastaut syndrome
Appears in the first year and is associated with cortical dysgenesis and mental impairment	Infantile spasms (West syndrome)
Associated with antibodies against glutamate receptors	Rasmussen encephalitis
Seizures that occur in response to particular stimuli	Reflex epilepsy

What is the inheritance pattern of benign childhood epilepsy?	Autosomal dominant
What is the long-term outlook in Lennox-Gastaut syndrome?	Seizures and intellectual impairment continue into adulthood.
To which hormones is West syndrome sometimes responsive?	Adrenocorticotropic hormone (ACTH) and corticosteroids
What surgical treatment is effective in severe unilateral Rasmussen encephalitis?	Partial hemispherectomy
What is the most common stimulus known to trigger reflex epilepsy?	Visual stimuli (especially television and video games)
What two mitochondrial disorders are associated with epilepsy syndromes?	MELAS (**M**itochondrial myopathy, **E**ncephalopathy, **L**actic **A**cidosis, and **S**troke episodes)
	MERRF (**M**yoclonic **E**pilepsy with **R**agged **R**ed **F**ibers)

What is the term used to describe a seizure that is not caused by abnormal firing of neurons, which is therefore unresponsive to antiepileptic drugs (AEDs)?	Psychogenic seizure
What features are usually missing in psychogenic seizures that help in differentiating them from actual seizures?	Tongue biting, incontinence, and postictal confusion/amnesia
What laboratory finding is useful in diagnosing a generalized seizure?	Elevated serum creatinine kinase
What is the likely cause of this increase in serum creatinine kinase?	Sustained muscle contraction

PATHOPHYSIOLOGY

What physiologic mechanisms probably underlie most seizure disorders?	Abnormally excitable neurons Increased glutamatergic neurotransmission Reduction in inhibitory GABA neurotransmission
What is the term used to describe the cellular interictal (between seizures) marker for epilepsy characterized by calcium-dependent depolarizations, which trigger sodium-mediated action potentials?	Paroxysmal depolarizing shift
What are the major genetic etiologies responsible for epileptic syndromes?	Channelopathies and cortical malformation
Which channels are commonly abnormal in channelopathies causing epilepsy?	Sodium, potassium, calcium, and $GABA_A$ chloride channel
What are some of the congenital diseases associated with both cortical malformation and epilepsy?	Holoprosencephaly, lissencephaly, double cortex, tuberous sclerosis, and Angelman syndrome
Withdrawal from which substances can result in seizures?	Alcohol, benzodiazepines, and barbiturates
What treatment is used to prevent seizures and delirium tremens during alcohol withdrawals?	Benzodiazepines

What condition is defined by hypertension and seizures during the third trimester of pregnancy? | Eclampsia

What therapies are available to treat eclampsia? | Magnesium infusion or caesarian section

ANTIEPILEPTIC DRUGS

What agents are indicated in the first-line treatment of both partial and tonic-clonic seizures? | Carbamazepine, phenytoin, and valproate

Which AED exhibits zero-order kinetics? | Phenytoin

What is meant by the term zero-order kinetics? | Clearance of the drug is fixed and not dependent on concentration.

What causes a drug to have zero-order kinetics? | Metabolic enzymes are saturated at concentrations below therapeutic range.

What are the side effects of phenytoin? | Gingival hyperplasia, coarsening of facial features, hirsutism, and teratogenicity (fetal hydantoin syndrome)

What is the mechanism of action (MOA) of phenytoin? | Binds to sodium channels in the inactive state

In which two scenarios would you be most likely to use phenytoin? | 1. Treatment of tonic-clonic seizures 2. Treatment of status epilepticus

How is fosphenytoin different than phenytoin? | Fosphenytoin is a prodrug (metabolizes to phenytoin) that is safer for parenteral administration.

What other AEDs function via blockade of sodium channels? | Carbamazepine, valproate, lamotrigine, and zonisamide

Which AEDs are associated with cytochrome p450 enzyme induction? | Carbamazepine, phenobarbital, and phenytoin

What other condition can carbamazepine be useful in treating? | Neuropathic pain

What rare hematologic complications are seen following use of carbamazepine? | Aplastic anemia and agranulocytosis

Which AED is associated with cytochrome p450 inhibition?	Valproate
What are the proposed MOAs of valproate?	Potentiation of GABA Blockade of repetitive firing Inhibition of calcium T-channels
Which of these mechanisms is most likely the cause for efficacy of valproate in absence seizures?	Inhibition of calcium T-channels
Why is phenobarbital preferred in the treatment of partial and tonic-clonic seizures during pregnancy?	Carbamazepine, phenytoin, and valproate are all teratogenic.
Why should valproate be avoided during pregnancy?	Predisposes to neural tube defects
Deficiency of which vitamin is responsible for neural tube defects?	Folate
What other side effects are associated with valproate?	Hepatotoxicity and weight gain
Which AEDs block glutamate receptors?	Topiramate blocks AMPA/kainite receptors and felbamate blocks NMDA.
What is the MOA of tiagabine?	Inhibits GABA reuptake
What is the MOA of vigabatrin?	Blocks GABA breakdown
Which AEDs may exacerbate absence seizures?	Tiagabine, vigabatrin, and gabapentin
What is the mechanism for exacerbation of absence seizures by these drugs?	Increased $GABA_B$ transmission
Which classes of AEDs act on the $GABA_A$ receptor?	Benzodiazepines and barbiturates
Which AEDs are contraindicated in porphyria?	Barbiturates
What nonpharmacologic therapies are used in the management of epilepsy?	Ketogenic diet Vagus nerve stimulation Surgical excision of foci (intractable cases) Corpus callosotomy Hemispherectomy (Rasmussen and Sturge-Weber)

CLINICAL VIGNETTES

Make the diagnosis for the following patients:

A 35-year-old woman recently began having complex partial seizures with olfactory auras—she reports smelling burning rubber. She had a febrile seizure as a child, but has had no other seizures in her life. MRI demonstrates medial temporal sclerosis.

Temporal lobe epilepsy

A 7-year-old boy is brought to the doctor because concerned teachers report excessive daydreaming, during which he is unresponsive. Staring spells also include blinking and eye rolling. On physical examination, an unresponsive staring spell is brought on by hyperventilation. EEG demonstrates 3-Hz spike and wave pattern.

Absence seizure

A 3-year-old boy is brought to the neurologist because he has had multiple types of seizures, and has failed to reach some developmental milestones. EEG demonstrates a slow 2-Hz spike and wave pattern.

Lennox-Gastaut syndrome

CHAPTER 14

Dementia and Degenerative Disease

MEMORY

What is the term used to describe the following types of memory?

Memory for things that can be verbally demonstrated

Explicit or declarative memory

Memory or learning that cannot be elucidated in precise terms

Implicit memory

Includes both skills and conditioning (classical and operant)

Implicit memory

Type of explicit memory specific to events and sequence in time

Episodic memory

Type of explicit memory specific to factual information

Semantic memory

Short-term recall of things for the purpose of mental processing and manipulation

Working memory

Associated with the prefrontal cortex with potential involvement of the cerebellum

Working memory

Type of memory usually defective in amnestic disorders

Episodic

What two structures are considered critical for memory?

1. Hippocampus
2. Medial thalamus nuclei (especially dorsomedial nucleus)

AMNESIA

What term is used to describe impaired ability to recall events prior to injury?	Retrograde amnesia
What is the term used to describe the inability to form new memory?	Anterograde amnesia
What is the amnestic disorder commonly seen in alcoholic patients?	Korsakoff syndrome (see Chap. 8 for more information)
What is the term used to describe a condition of amnesia for present and recent events and confusion lasting hours?	Transient global amnesia
What is the only memory deficit seen after recovery from transient global amnesia?	Only loss of memory for the period of the attack

DEMENTIA

List some of the neurologic consequences of normal aging:	Presbyopia Diminished night vision Presbycusis Diminished olfaction Reduced motor activity and speed Reduced reflexes Loss of vibration sense
What is the term used to describe the deterioration of cognitive function without alteration of consciousness or perception?	Dementia
What is the term used to describe a confusional state involving altered consciousness, perception, and a hyperreactive state?	Delirium
What reversible causes need to be investigated in a patient with suspected dementia?	Hypothyroidism Vitamin deficiency Depression Syphilis Structural lesions

How should a clinician differentiate between depression (pseudodementia) and true dementia?	Depression screening and interview family member
Which patients are more likely to report a deficit?	Depressed patients will report deficits, while demented patients are more likely to attempt to hide deficits.
What is the term used to describe the prodromal intellectual impairment that precedes progression to dementia?	Mild cognitive impairment (MCI)
What is the most common cause of dementia?	Alzheimer disease (AD)
What are the earliest signs of AD?	Gradual forgetfulness and difficulty with numbers
With what complaints do patients with AD initially present?	Vague dizziness, fogginess, or nondescript headache
What cognitive functions are most severely affected by AD?	Memory, language, and mathematics
What later deficits occur in the "executive functions" attributed to the frontal lobes?	Inattention Impaired judgment Mental inflexibility Perseveration (making same mistakes)
What are some of the latest symptoms in AD?	Loss of social graces, paranoia, and hallucinations
Which memories are the earliest to be lost in dementing illnesses?	Recent memories
What is the term used to describe nighttime confusion, restlessness, and inversion of sleep pattern that occurs in dementia?	Sundowning
What is the prognosis associated with AD?	Patients usually succumb to infections, particularly pneumonia about 10 years from diagnosis.
What regions of the brain are typically involved in the diffuse neuronal loss associated with AD?	Hippocampus, association cortex of the frontal, temporal, and parietal lobes, and the cholinergic nucleus basalis of Meynert

What is the rationale for cholinergic therapies such as cholinergic agonists and cholinesterase inhibitors?

Counteract the loss of cholinergic projections from the basal forebrain

What are the three microscopic components of AD pathology?

1. Neurofibrillary tangles
2. Senile or neuritic plaques
3. Granulovacuolar degeneration

What microtubule-associated protein is the primary component of neurofibrillary tangles?

Tau

What post-translational modification of tau may lead to altered conformation, paired helical filament formation, and neurofibrillary tangle deposition?

Hyperphosphorylation

What is the primary component of senile plaques?

Amyloid beta (Aβ)

What is meant by the term amyloid?

Protein with predominantly beta-sheet conformation that forms extracellular deposits

What are the characteristic properties of amyloid?

Staining with Congo red dye and apple green birefringence

Amyloid derived from which proteins are described as primary amyloidosis?

Immunoglobulins

What genes, associated with familial forms of AD, code for components of the gamma-secretase complex involved in processing amyloid precursor protein (APP) into Aβ?

Presenilin 1 and 2

What is thought to be the reason for early-onset AD in trisomy 21?

Excess copies of APP gene located on chromosome 21

What lipoprotein allele is associated with late-onset AD?

ApoE4

What finding can be seen on brain imaging in AD patients?

Enlargement of third and lateral ventricles due to neuronal degeneration

A newer drug used in the treatment of AD, memantine, is an antagonist of which receptor?

N-methyl-D-aspartate (NMDA)-type glutamate receptor

What type of dementia is seen in patients with a history of stroke, hypertension, and may be seen in combination with AD?	Vascular dementia
What type of vascular dementia is the second most common cause of dementia after AD?	Multiinfarct dementia
What vascular dementia caused by persistent hypertension causes lacunar infarcts and subcortical demyelination?	Binswanger disease
Which dementing illness can be clinically distinguished from AD by the presence of visual hallucinations and parkinsonism?	Dementia with Lewy bodies (DLB)
What is the major protein component of a Lewy body?	α-Synuclein
What other neurodegenerative disease includes Lewy bodies as part of its pathology?	Parkinson disease (PD)
What term is used to encompass both dementia from diffuse frontal lobe degeneration as well as an aphasic syndrome known as primary progressive aphasia?	Frontotemporal dementia (FTD)
What is the typical presentation of a patient with the frontal lobe dementia form of FTD?	Alterations in personality and social conduct in an elderly individual
Describe the defect seen in patients with primary progressive aphasia:	Difficulty with word-finding (anomia) progresses to a global language problem.
How is the pathology of FTD similar to AD?	Diffuse neuronal loss and tau deposition
What is the specific form of FTD in which pathology includes swollen neurons and argentophilic bodies?	Pick disease (Pick bodies)
What is the prognosis for Pick disease?	2–5-year survival
What rapidly progressive dementing illness with myoclonus is associated with prions?	Creutzfeldt-Jakob disease (CJD)

What is the typical survival time after diagnosis of CJD?	<1 year
Immunoassay for what protein is used in diagnostic testing for CJD?	14-3-3
What are some of the iatrogenic sources of CJD?	Corneal transplants Dural grafts Human gonadotropins and growth hormone (GH) EEG depth electrodes

OTHER NEURODEGENERATIVE DISEASE

What autosomal dominant disease causes choreoathetosis and dementia?	Huntington disease (HD)
What is the genetic alteration responsible for HD?	Triplet repeat (CAG) expansion of the huntingtin gene (>40 copies) resulting in a polyglutamine motif
What is the term used to describe the earlier onset and increased severity due to repeat expansion in subsequent generations?	Anticipation
What is the location of the huntingtin gene?	Short arm of chromosome 4
What structures are subject to severe degenerative atrophy causing hydrocephalus ex vacuo?	Head of caudate nucleus
What is the typical survival time for patients with HD from the time of diagnosis?	15–20 years
What neurodegenerative disease affecting nearly 1% of the elderly population causes bradykinesia, resting tremor, and cogwheel rigidity?	Parkinson disease (PD)
Loss of >80% of which group of dopaminergic neurons is responsible for PD?	Substantia nigra pars compacta (see Chap. 7 for more information regarding PD)
Insidious onset of disequilibrium, falls, visual problems, and personality change in one's sixties are suggestive of what tau-related disease?	Progressive supranuclear palsy (PSP)

What are the primary consequences of PSP?	Supranuclear ophthalmoplegia and pseudobulbar palsy
What autosomal recessive triplet repeat disease is the most common etiology of hereditary ataxia?	Friedrich ataxia
What is the name of the gene on chromosome 9 whose expression is suppressed by GAA repeat expansion in Friedrich ataxia?	Frataxin
What is the typical age of onset of Friedrich ataxia?	Early adolescence
What are the main features of Friedrich ataxia?	Ataxia and gait disorder Cardiomyopathy Kyphoscoliosis
What other disorders are associated with the foot deformity known as *pes cavus* seen in Friedrich ataxia?	Charcot-Marie-Tooth and muscular dystrophy
What disease of upper and lower motor neurons presents with weakness in distal extremities and atrophy of the hands and forearms, but no sensory alterations?	Amyotrophic lateral sclerosis (ALS) (aka Lou Gehrig disease)
What is the typical survival time of a patient with ALS from time of diagnosis?	3–6 years
A familial form of ALS is associated with a deficiency of which free radical neutralizing enzyme?	Cu/Zn-superoxide dismutase (SOD1)

CLINICAL VIGNETTES

Make the diagnosis for the following patients:

A wife brings her 62-year-old husband to a neurologist because his behavior has drastically changed over the last few months. He neglects matters of personal hygiene, including bathing and shaving. He has been uncharacteristically using profanity and making inappropriate sexual comments in social settings, and is aggressive at times. Mental status examination reveals normal memory function, but some language difficulty, particularly with word finding. MRI of the brain reveals marked cerebral atrophy of the frontal and temporal lobes with no masses. Autopsy findings include gliosis, swollen neurons, and argentophilic bodies.

Pick disease—form of frontotemporal dementia

A 70-year-old retired electrical engineer has an insidious onset of forgetfulness, difficulty concentrating, and personality changes. He has no history of hypertension (HTN) or cerebrovascular disease. Physical examination is unremarkable for focal neurologic signs or signs of depression. On mental status examination, he is unable to perform certain math problems and can only recall one out of three items after 5 minutes. His mini-mental score was 17. Liver function tests (LFTs) are normal, thyroid-stimulating hormone (TSH) and cortisol levels were normal, rapid plasma reagent (RPR) was negative, and cobalamin levels were normal. MRI of the brain reveals diffuse cortical atrophy. Autopsy findings include senile plaques and neurofibrillary tangles.

Alzheimer disease

A 60-year-old male is brought to the ER because he was found stumbling and acting in a bizarre manner. His breath smells strongly of alcohol, and he appears homeless. On physical examination, he exhibits ataxia and nystagmus, and recalls only one out of four items in the mini-mental status examination.

Wernicke-Korsakoff encephalopathy

CHAPTER 15

Congenital Disorders

MENTAL RETARDATION

What is the most common cause of mental retardation?	Fetal alcohol syndrome (FAS) (about 1:750 live births)
What are the common problems associated with FAS?	Congenital heart disease, microcephaly, limb dislocation, facial abnormalities, and holoprosencephaly (if severe)
What facial abnormalities are seen in FAS?	Short palpebral fissure, epicanthal folds, and flat philtrum/midface hypoplasia
What is the most common cause of inherited mental retardation?	Fragile X syndrome
What physical features are associated with fragile X syndrome?	Large ears, prominent jaw, long narrow face, and macroorchidism (large testes)
What is the genetic defect in fragile X syndrome?	Triplet repeat disorder (CGG) in *FMR1* gene
What developmental disorder is commonly associated with fragile X syndrome?	Autism
What defects are most common in autism?	Lack of social and communication skills and repetitive ritualistic behaviors
What is the term used to describe a high functioning form of autism often associated with savant features?	Asperger syndrome
Besides fragile X syndrome, what X-linked genetic disease is associated with autism?	Rett syndrome

What characteristic repetitive motor behavior is often seen in Rett syndrome?	Hand-wringing
Why is Rett syndrome only seen in females?	Embryonic lethality in males due to single X chromosome
What is the most common autosomal chromosome abnormality that causes mental retardation?	Trisomy 21 (Down syndrome) (about 1:800 live births)
What is the most common cause of trisomy 21?	Nondisjunction (95% of all cases)
What is the most common cause of trisomy 21 in a patient with 46 chromosomes?	Robertsonian translocation (4% of all cases)
What abnormality in maternal serum alpha-fetoprotein (AFP) is seen in Down syndrome?	Decreased AFP
What is the characteristic appearance of trisomy 21?	Flattened face, dysplastic ears, protruding tongue, microcephaly, epicanthal folds, upward slanting palpebral fissures, and simian crease
What are the medical problems associated with trisomy 21?	Acute lymphoblastic and myeloid leukemias, septum primum atrial septal defect (ASD), duodenal atresia, and early onset Alzheimer disease (about age 35)
What syndrome presents with mental retardation, decreased muscle tone, emotional lability, and obesity?	Prader-Willi syndrome
What is the genetic defect in Prader-Willi syndrome?	Deletion of imprinted region of paternal 15q11-13 locus
What syndrome presents with mental retardation, abnormal gait, seizures, and inappropriate happy behavior?	Angelman syndrome (happy puppet syndrome)
What is the genetic defect in Angelman syndrome?	Deletion of imprinted region of maternal 15q11-13 locus
Define genomic imprinting:	Genes are expressed differently based on parental origin. For example, Prader-Willi syndrome results from deletion of important paternal genes on chromosome 15 which are not actively expressed from the maternal chromosome.

| What is the mechanism behind genomic imprinting? | Differential DNA methylation at cytosine bases prevents expression of genes from either the maternal or paternal chromosome. For example, methylation of the maternal chromosome prevents active expression of the genes missing from the paternal chromosome in Prader-Willi syndrome. |

CONGENITAL ANOMALIES

What is the term used to describe the following developmental defects:

Failure of midline cleavage of the prosencephalon	Holoprosencephaly
Congenital lack of the gyri and sulci of the brain	Lissencephaly, or "smooth brain"
Neuromigrational disorder that produces a cerebrospinal fluid (CSF)-filled cleft along the surface of the entire cortex	Schizencephaly, or "split brain"
Congenital cranial herniation	Encephalocele
Premature fusion of the cranial sutures	Craniosynostosis

With which diseases is holoprosencephaly associated?	Trisomy 13 (Patau syndrome) and severe FAS
What is the characteristic facial appearance of holoprosencephaly?	Cyclopia, cleft lip and palate, and hypotelorism
What underlying signaling pathway may be defective in holoprosencephaly?	Sonic Hedgehog (SHH) signaling
What are the main causes of craniosynostosis?	Abnormal ossification of the skull (primary craniosynostosis), or more commonly, a failure in brain growth (secondary craniosynostosis)
What congenital disease is due to a defect in the occipital bone?	Cranium bifidum
What problems are associated with cranium bifidum?	Herniation of meninges and cerebellar tissue
What disease is caused by failure of the anterior neuropore to close?	Anencephaly

What problem in pregnancy is associated with anencephaly? — Polyhydramnios

What disease is caused by a failure of posterior neuropore closure? — Spina bifida (incomplete spinal closure)

What lab result is commonly seen in neural tube defects? — Increased AFP

What is the common dietary problem leading to neural tube defects? — Insufficient folic acid in the maternal diet

Which form of spina bifida offers no clinical findings? — Spina bifida occulta

Which form of spina bifida produces herniated meninges? — Spina bifida cystica

What are the two main types of herniations in spina bifida cystica? —
1. Meningocele (meninges only)
2. Meningomyelocele (spinal cord and meninges)

A thoracolumbar meningomyelocele is often part of what malformation? — Arnold-Chiari malformation type II (ACM II)

What is an Arnold-Chiari malformation type I (ACM I)? — Cerebellar tonsils and medulla herniate through the foramen magnum

What are the classic findings of an ACM? — Elongation of the cerebellar tonsils, beaking of the colliculi, and thickening of the upper cervical spinal cord

What name is given to the abnormally curved appearance of the cerebellum on sonogram? — Banana sign

What medical problems are ACM I associated with? — Hydrocephalus, syringomyelia, and spina bifida

How is ACM II unique from ACM I? — Includes a thoracolumbar meningomyelocele (plus all findings of ACM I)

What is a Dandy-Walker malformation? — Triad: (1) agenesis or hypoplasia of the cerebellar vermis, (2) cystic dilation of the fourth ventricle, and (3) an enlargement of the posterior fossa

What is the most common mechanism behind congenital hydrocephalus? — Aqueduct stenosis

What physical examination finding is seen in babies with hydrocephalus, but not adults?	Large heads (Their skulls are still expandable and soft.)
What causes a large head in kids when the amount of CSF is normal?	Hydranencephaly
What causes hydranencephaly?	Bilateral internal carotid artery occlusion in utero (causes a near-total absence of cerebral cortex and basal ganglia)
What is the most common movement disorder in children?	Cerebral palsy (CP)
What is the most common form of CP?	Spastic or pyramidal CP
What causes CP?	Fixed (nonprogressive) lesion of the immature brain, especially the motor tracts
What is the most common cause of intracranial hemorrhage in kids?	Arteriovenous malformation (AVM)
How can you check for an AVM on physical examination of a newborn?	Auscultate for a cranial bruit

GENETIC DEFECTS

What disease results in mental retardation and growth retardation when mothers consume the artificial sweetener aspartame?	Maternal phenylketonuria (PKU)
What is the defect in PKU?	A lack of phenylalanine hydroxylase
What is the treatment for PKU?	Dietary: avoid phenylalanine and supplement with tyrosine
What disease presents in early childhood with proximal muscle weakness?	Duchenne muscular dystrophy (DMD)
What early clinical signs suggest DMD in a child?	Hypertrophied calves and Gower sign
What is Gower sign?	Using the arms to rise from a seat
What is the genetic defect of DMD?	X-linked recessive frameshift mutation leading to deletion of the dystrophin gene

What disease is a milder form of DMD?	Becker muscular dystrophy (dystrophin gene is only mutated)
What inherited disease is caused by degeneration of the anterior horn cells and cranial nerve motor nuclei?	Spinal muscle atrophy (aka Werdnig-Hoffman disease)
How does spinal muscle atrophy present?	Generalized motor weakness and hypotonia
What disease classically presents with cerebellar dysfunction, spider angiomata, and no IgA?	Ataxia-telangiectasia
What is the underlying defect in ataxia-telangiectasia?	Autosomal recessive defect in DNA repair enzyme

LYSOSOMAL STORAGE DISEASES

What are the main neural consequences of lysosomal storage disease?	Peripheral neuropathy (Krabbe disease, Fabry disease), progressive neurodegeneration (Tay-Sachs disease, Niemann-Pick disease), or demyelination (metachromatic leukodystrophy)
What disease is suspected in a patient with a cherry-red spot on the macula, hepatosplenomegaly, and progressive neurodegeneration?	Niemann-Pick disease
What physical finding helps differentiate Tay-Sachs from Niemann-Pick disease?	Only Niemann-Pick disease shows hepatosplenomegaly.
What is the enzyme deficiency associated with Niemann-Pick disease?	Sphingomyelinase, leading to excess sphingomyelin
What disease is suspected in a patient with hepatosplenomegaly, mental retardation, and bone pain?	Gaucher disease
What is the enzyme deficiency associated with Gaucher disease?	β-Glucocerebrosidase, leading to excess glucocerebroside
What pathologic finding is characteristic of Gaucher disease?	Gaucher cells, which are macrophages with "crinkled paper" cytoplasm (light microscopy)

What is the enzyme deficiency associated with Tay-Sachs disease?

Hexosaminidase A, leading to excess GM2 ganglioside

What pathologic finding is characteristic of Tay-Sachs disease?

Lysozymes with whorled configurations of membranes inside (electron microscopy)

What disease is associated with coarse facial features, severe neurologic degeneration, and corneal clouding?

Hurler syndrome

What is the enzyme deficiency associated with Hurler syndrome?

α-L-Iduronidase, leading to excess heparin sulfate and dermatan sulfate

Which disease is similar to Hurler syndrome clinically, but has a different pathophysiology?

I-Cell disease

What is the defect involved in I-Cell disease?

Failure to add mannose-6-phosphate to lysosome proteins

What disease presents as a milder form of Hurler syndrome?

Hunter syndrome

What is the enzyme deficiency associated with Hunter syndrome?

Iduronate sulfatase, leading to too much heparin sulfate and dermatan sulfate

How is the presentation of Hunter syndrome distinct from Hurler syndrome?

No corneal clouding and an aggressive personality in Hunter syndrome

MITOCHONDRIAL DISEASES

What mitochondrial disease presents with bilateral visual loss in the teenage years?

LHON (Leber hereditary optic neuropathy)

What mitochondrial disease presents with ataxia, myopathy, and seizures?

MERRF (Myoclonic Epilepsy with Ragged Red Fibers)

What mitochondrial disease presents with stroke-like episodes and lactic acidosis?

MELAS (Mitochondrial Encephalomyopathy, Lactic Acidosis, Stroke-like episodes)

What mitochondrial disease presents with loss of developmental milestones, hypotonia, and choreoathetoid hand movements?

Leigh subacute necrotizing encephalomyopathy (Leigh disease)

What are the unifying characteristics of all genetic mitochondrial diseases?

Heteroplasmy and maternal inheritance

Define heteroplasmy:

Variation of phenotype related to the number of mitochondria affected

CLINICAL VIGNETTES

Make the diagnosis for the following patients:

A 4-year-old female is brought to your office by her concerned parents. They report that she has always walked funny. They have grown concerned because she never grew out of it, and in fact, it has become steadily worse. Physical examination reveals red "spider-looking" veins on her cheek and at the corner of her eyes, wide-based and unsteady gait, and dysarthric speech. Optokinetic nystagmus is absent and she turns her head rather than her eyes when shifting gaze. Blood tests reveal a low lymphocyte count and decreased IgA levels. MRI reveals mild cerebellar atrophy with an enlarged fourth ventricle.

Ataxia telangiectasia

A 35-year-old male with history of HTN, cardiomyopathy, scoliosis, and obesity presents with slowly progressing difficulty jogging and lately, trouble getting out of bed without using his arms. He has noticed his calves are enlarged. Physical examination reveals deep tendon reflexes are 1+ throughout, strength decreased in lower extremity more than upper extremity. Laboratory studies demonstrate moderately elevated CPK. On muscle biopsy, staining shows dystrophin to be fragmented and patchy.

Becker muscular dystrophy

A 10-year-old girl with no significant PMH presents with headache, neck pain, and difficulty walking. Her parents first noticed problems when she burned her hand on a stove without pulling her hand away or showing concern. Physical examination demonstrates ataxic gait, with normal strength and reflexes, and decreased pain and temperature sensation in the upper extremities. Ophthalmoscopic examination reveals bilateral papilledema. CT scan reveals peg-like cerebellar tonsils, a thick upper cervical cord, and hydrocephalus.

Arnold-Chiari malformation I

A 35-year-old G2P2 female with known bipolar disorder recently gave birth to a 38-week-old girl via spontaneous vaginal delivery. During her pregnancy, she experienced periods of mania and was compelled to stay on her medication. Her child experienced no obvious symptoms. Physical examination reveals a small patch of hair at the base of the spine. X-ray revealed bony abnormalities at L5 and S1.

Spina bifida occulta

A healthy 28-year-old G1P1 female gave birth to a male child 1 year ago, who was found to have some dysmorphic features. The child was found to have a long narrow face with large ears and a prominent jaw. Testicular examination revealed larger than expected testicles bilaterally, which have remained enlarged. Genetic testing revealed an increased number of CGG repeats. The child has been nonresponsive to his mother's attention, preferring instead to stare at his bottle for long periods of time.

Fragile X syndrome

CHAPTER 16

Nutritional and Metabolic Disease

What are some of the most common causes of nutritional deficiencies?	Alcoholism, celiac sprue, pernicious anemia, and gastrointestinal (GI) resection
Which syndromes are seen as a consequence of thiamine (vitamin B$_1$) deficiency?	Wernicke-Korsakoff syndrome and beriberi
How does alcohol contribute to deficiency?	Chronic alcoholism leads to decreased thiamine uptake, storage, and utilization.
Administration of dextrose to unconscious patients without what other agent can precipitate or exacerbate Wernicke encephalopathy?	Thiamine
What are the symptoms of Wernicke encephalopathy?	Mental confusion, nystagmus, gaze palsy, and gait ataxia
What deficit seen in thiamine deficiency is referred to as Korsakoff syndrome?	Anterograde amnesia with confabulation (see Chap. 8 for more information on Wernicke-Korsakoff syndrome)
What are the primary manifestations of beriberi?	Peripheral neuropathy and cardiac pathology
What symptoms make wet beriberi different from dry beriberi?	Edema and high output congestive heart failure (CHF)
What are the symptoms of the peripheral neuropathy seen with beriberi?	Weakness, paresthesias, and pain
What is the term used to describe niacin deficiency resulting in a triad of dementia, dermatitis, and diarrhea?	Pellagra

What other symptom is occasionally seen in pellagra?	Glossitis
What amino acid is the precursor of niacin synthesis?	Tryptophan
Diets based primarily on what vegetable tend to be deficient in tryptophan and niacin?	Corn
What disease of defective transport of neutral amino acids across the renal tubule can cause symptoms of pellagra?	Hartnup disease
What vitamin deficiency can lead to degeneration of the dorsal and lateral columns of the spinal cord, known as subacute combined degeneration?	Vitamin B_{12} (cobalamin)
What is the most consistent pattern of sensory loss seen in subacute combined degeneration?	Loss of vibration sense
Damage to which descending spinal tract causes progressive weakness in subacute combined degeneration?	Lateral corticospinal tract
What hematologic findings result from vitamin B_{12} deficiency?	Megaloblastic anemia and hypersegmented neutrophils
What is the term used to describe a deficiency of vitamin B_{12} due to lack of intrinsic factor?	Pernicious anemia
What other malabsorption syndromes cause vitamin B_{12} deficiency?	Celiac sprue, GI resection, blind loop syndrome, *Diphyllobothrium latum* (fish tapeworm), Crohn disease, and atrophic gastritis
Alterations in the myelin sheath resulting from vitamin B_{12} deficiency are believed to be caused by accumulation of what molecule?	Methylmalonyl CoA
What vitamin deficiency associated with isoniazid treatment leads to paresthesias and in severe cases, seizures?	Pyridoxine (vitamin B_6)
Deficiency of what lipid-soluble antioxidant vitamin can sometimes cause spinocerebellar degeneration and ataxia?	Vitamin E (tocopherol)

Deficiency of what lipid-soluble vitamin leads to night blindness, follicular keratosis, and dry corneas?	Vitamin A (retinoic acid)
What conditions prevent the absorption of lipid-soluble vitamins?	Cystic fibrosis, sprue, pancreatic insufficiency, inflammatory bowel disease, cholestasis, bacterial overgrowth, and some GI resections
What are the consequences of vitamin A excess?	Headache, alopecia, rash, and in severe cases pseudotumor cerebri
Consumption of which organ can lead to excess vitamin A?	Liver (notably polar bear liver)
Degeneration of which brain region in chronic alcoholism leads to ataxia, wide-based gait, and intention tremor?	Cerebellar vermis
What is the name of the disease, mostly seen in alcoholics, resulting in degeneration of the corpus callosum and anterior commissure?	Marchiafava-Bignami disease
What gas, produced by home furnaces, has a much greater affinity for hemoglobin than oxygen?	Carbon monoxide
What are the symptoms of carbon monoxide poisoning?	Headache, nausea, confusion, and dizziness
What is the site of lesions resulting from carbon monoxide poisoning?	Globus pallidus
What device is incapable of accurately measuring oxygen saturation in presence of carbon monoxide poisoning?	Pulse oximeter
If you suspect carbon monoxide poisoning, what test should you get instead?	Arterial blood gas
How is oxygen saturation restored in cases of carbon monoxide poisoning?	Hyperbaric oxygen
At what blood glucose do patients typically start to exhibit symptoms of hypoglycemia?	30 mg/dL
What division of the nervous system is responsible for the agitation, flushing, sweating, and palpitations that occur during hypoglycemia?	Sympathetic nervous system

What feature of diabetic neuropathy can interfere with the sympathetic response to hypoglycemia?	Autonomic dysfunction
What symptoms follow sympathetic signs of hypoglycemia?	Confusion, drowsiness, and seizures
What biochemical changes are believed to be responsible for hypoglycemic convulsions?	Increased ammonium and decreased gamma-aminobutyric acid (GABA)
What are the most likely causes of severe hypoglycemia?	Insulin overdose and insulinoma
What test could be used to distinguish between excess insulin administration and insulinoma?	C peptide (elevated in insulinoma, normal in insulin overdose)
At what blood glucose level is a hypoglycemic patient likely to enter a comatose state?	10 mg/dL
What potentially lethal complication of type 1 diabetes mellitus can result from low insulin?	Diabetic ketoacidosis (DKA)
What is the term used to describe the abnormal breathing pattern during DKA?	Kussmaul breathing (deep rapid breath; described as air hunger)
What changes will be observed in arterial blood gases of a patient exhibiting Kussmaul breathing?	Low CO_2
What laboratory findings are associated with DKA?	Ketones, β-hydroxybutyrate, and glucose in urine
What is the term used to describe the coma induced by hyperglycemia in type 2 diabetics?	Hyperosmolar nonketotic coma
What treatment is indicated for both DKA and hyperosmolar nonketotic coma?	Intravenous fluids and insulin
At what blood glucose level do patients run an increased risk of hyperosmolar nonketotic coma?	600 mg/dL
What is the term used to describe clonic movement on extension of the hands in patients with hepatic encephalopathy?	Asterixis

Which cells in the brain increase in number in order to handle the extra ammonium resulting from liver failure?

Astrocytes

What are the three major theories regarding the mechanism of hepatic encephalopathy?

1. Ammonium toxicity
2. False neurotransmitter
3. GABA-benzodiazepine

CLINICAL VIGNETTES

Make the diagnosis for the following patients:

A 45-year-old Inuit male complains of recent onset of headache, hair loss, and skin rash. He recently returned from hunting big game, including polar bears. Physical examination reveals skin discoloration on the palms and soles and papilledema.

Vitamin A excess

A 25-year-old female is brought to the ER by a friend after having a seizure. The friend reports she seemed agitated and was flushed, sweating, and complained of weakness and palpitations prior to the seizure. She has no history of diabetes. Laboratory studies found blood glucose of 25 mg/dL and severely elevated C-peptide.

Insulinoma

CHAPTER 17

Peripheral Neuropathy

Which cranial nerves are not considered part of the peripheral nervous system?	Olfactory and optic nerves (CN I and II)
What are the connective tissue layers of peripheral nerves from outermost to innermost?	Epineurium Perineurium Endoneurium
Which connective tissue layer is continuous with the dura mater?	Epineurium
Suturing of which connective tissue layer is used in repair of severed peripheral nerves?	Epineurium
What is the term used to describe the following?	
Peripheral nerve pathology with myelin degeneration and axon sparing	Segmental demyelination
Peripheral nerve pathology with anterograde degeneration of both myelin and the axon distal to the site of injury	Wallerian degeneration
Dying back process that occurs as a result of metabolic polyneuropathy	Axonal degeneration
Swelling, peripheral nucleus, and loss of Nissl substance as a result of axonal injury	Chromatolysis
Homogeneous clustering of muscle fiber pattern seen following nerve injury and reinnervation	Type grouping
Painful aberrant nodular growth of damaged cutaneous nerves	Traumatic or pseudoneuromas

Name the type of peripheral neuropathy described below:

Peripheral neuropathy resulting in symmetric weakness or paralysis progressing in an axon length–dependent manner

Polyneuropathy

Pain and sensory or motor loss in the distribution of a spinal nerve root

Radiculopathy

Motor or sensory deficit as a result of damage to anterior horn or ganglion cells

Neuronopathy

Motor or sensory deficit in the distribution of a single peripheral nerve

Mononeuropathy

Motor or sensory deficit due to injury to a peripheral nerve plexus

Plexopathy

What cause of ascending paralysis is often preceded by respiratory or GI illness?

Guillain-Barré syndrome (see Chap. 12)

What pseudomembrane-forming bacterium is also associated with a Guillain-Barré syndrome–like peripheral neuropathy?

Corynebacterium diphtheriae

What cellular process is inhibited by the diphtheria exotoxin associated with cranial and polyneuropathy?

Protein synthesis

Which mycobacterial infection causes a symmetrical polyneuropathy?

Leprosy

What tick-borne disease should be suspected in cases of bilateral facial nerve palsy?

Lyme disease

What is the causative agent of Lyme disease?

Borrelia burgdorferi

What are the possible symptoms of facial nerve palsy (Bell palsy)?

Paralysis of muscles of facial expression

Loss of taste on anterior 2/3 of tongue

Hyperacusis

Decreased lacrimation and salivation

What cranial nerve problem is associated with idiopathic unilateral facial pain in the V2 and V3 divisions?

Trigeminal neuralgia (tic douloureux)

What disease associated with dark urine causes motor polyneuropathy, abdominal pain, and psychosis?	Acute intermittent porphyria
What by-products of heme synthesis are found in the urine of patients with acute intermittent porphyria?	Amino-levulinic acid and porphobilinogen
Anti-Hu antibodies cause peripheral neuropathy as a paraneoplastic syndrome of which lung carcinoma?	Small cell lung cancer
Which diseases of excess immunoglobulin are associated with peripheral neuropathy due to amyloid deposition and antimyelin antibodies?	Multiple myeloma, Waldenström macroglobulinemia, and plasmacytoma
What is the term used to describe an apical lung tumor that causes a compression mononeuropathy, brachial plexopathy, and occasionally Horner syndrome?	Pancoast tumor
Which antineoplastic drugs, acting on microtubules, are associated with peripheral neuropathy?	Paclitaxel and vincristine
What platinum-containing antineoplastic agents cause damage to the dorsal columns?	Cisplatin and carboplatin
What antituberculosis drug causes a peripheral neuropathy due to pyridoxine deficiency?	Isoniazid (INH)
What drug used to treat bladder infections and associated with rust-colored or brown urine can cause peripheral neuropathy?	Nitrofurantoin
What is the most common cause of polyneuropathy?	Diabetes mellitus
What percentage of diabetics show evidence of peripheral neuropathy after 25 years with the disease?	About 50%
What are the main types of peripheral neuropathy seen in diabetic patients?	Symmetric sensory polyneuropathy, oculomotor ophthalmoplegia, and autonomic neuropathy
What is the mechanism of nerve damage in diabetes mellitus?	Microvascular ischemia of *vasa nervorum*

In which region of the body do diabetics first experience numbness and tingling?	Feet followed by hands
What is the term used to describe the length-dependent distribution of the symmetric polyneuropathy seen in diabetics?	Stocking and glove
What function is spared in the oculomotor ophthalmoplegia of diabetics?	Pupillary reflex
What are common features of autonomic neuropathy in diabetic patients?	Impotence, postural hypotension, bladder dysfunction, and gastroparesis
What is the only means of preventing diabetic neuropathy?	Tight glycemic control
What drugs, sometimes used for neuropathic pain, may help in the treatment of paresthesias due to polyneuropathy?	Antiepileptic drugs (AEDs) and antidepressants
What type of disease is associated with combinations of mononeuropathy, known as mononeuropathy multiplex?	Vasculitis

Name the vasculitides associated with the following:

Glomerulonephritis, lung hemorrhage, and P-ANCA antibodies	Polyarteritis nodosa (PAN)
Asthma, sinusitis, hypereosinophilia, and C-ANCA	Churg-Strauss syndrome
Granulomas of lungs and kidneys, saddlenose deformity, and C-ANCA	Wegener granulomatosis
Keratoconjunctivitis sicca and xerostomia	Sjögren syndrome
What is the most common disease of inherited peripheral neuropathy?	Charcot-Marie-Tooth disease (CMT)
What is the other name used to describe most forms of CMT disease?	Hereditary sensory and motor neuropathy (HSMN)
What is the typical age of onset for CMT?	Late childhood to adolescence

What are the physical signs of CMT disease?	Distal muscle weakness, calf atrophy, and pes cavus
What term is used to describe the thickening of peripheral nerves, palpable in some cases, due to demyelination and remyelination seen in CMT?	Onion-bulb

Name the other inherited causes of peripheral neuropathy associated with the following:

Arylsulfatase deficiency	Metachromatic leukodystrophy
α-Galactosidase deficiency and angiokeratomas	Fabry disease
β-Galactosidase deficiency and optic atrophy	Krabbe disease
Enlarged yellow-orange colored tonsils	Tangier disease

What is the term used to describe dermatomal radicular pain due to herpes zoster?	Shingles
What is the term used to describe herpes zoster that affects the geniculate ganglion and facial nerve?	Ramsey-Hunt syndrome
What spinal nerve roots contribute to the brachial plexus?	C5-T1

Name the nerve lesions associated with the following:

Damage to C5-C6 roots and waiter's tip position	Erb-Duchenne palsy
Injury to the lower brachial plexus and clawhand deformity	Klumpke paralysis
Cervical rib compressing the brachial plexus and subclavian vessels	Thoracic outlet syndrome
Wrist drop and alcoholism	Radial nerve palsy
Entrapment of the median nerve and excessive hand use	Carpal tunnel syndrome
Obesity, tight belts, and entrapment of the lateral femoral cutaneous nerve	Meralgia paresthetica

CLINICAL VIGNETTES

Make the diagnosis for the following patients:

A 55-year-old male with a 25-year history of type 2 diabetes complains of tingling and numbness in his feet and toes, worse at night, and recent erectile dysfunction. He does not perform regular fingerstick glucose tests. Physical examination demonstrates decreased response to microfilament, loss of vibratory sense, and HbA1c of 9.5.

Diabetic neuropathy

A 24-year-old man presents to the ER with bilateral facial paralysis. He reports having noticed a bull's eye rash after returning from camping. He also complains of recent onset of knee pain. On physical examination, the patient has erythema migrans and flaccid paralysis of facial muscles.

Lyme disease

A 45-year-old male is brought to the ER by his wife who explains that her husband has been experiencing excruciating abdominal pain, weakness, and is acting bizarrely. She reports that he recently began taking erythromycin for a bacterial infection. Urine from the patient turns dark while waiting to be processed by the lab, and is found to contain porphobilinogen.

Porphyria

A 55-year-old female with a history of asthma and sinusitis complains of recent foot drop and numbness in her leg. She reports exacerbation of asthma after discontinuing use of inhaled steroids. On physical examination, patient has wheezing, sensory loss in multiple nerve territories, nasal polyps, and hypereosinophilia.

Churg-Strauss syndrome

CHAPTER 18

Neuropharmacology

ANXIOLYTICS AND HYPNOTICS

What amino acid derivative serves as the central nervous system's (CNS) inhibitory neurotransmitter?

Gamma-aminobutyric acid (GABA)

What are the effects of benzodiazepines and barbiturates on the CNS?

Dose-dependent CNS depression

What are the different levels of CNS depression?

Anxiolysis, sedation, hypnosis, medullary depression, coma, and death

What is the mechanism of action of benzodiazepines?

Increased frequency of GABAergic chloride ion conductance

What is the mechanism of action of barbiturates?

Increased duration of GABAergic chloride ion conductance

Why are benzodiazepines generally safer than barbiturates?

Barbiturate overdose is lethal, whereas benzodiazepines exhibit indirect inhibition of the $GABA_A$ at high doses.

What pharmacokinetic properties determine the clinical utility of specific benzodiazepines and barbiturates?

Duration of onset and duration of action

Why are alprazolam, clonazepam, diazepam, and lorazepam the preferred benzodiazepines used in the treatment of anxiety disorders?

Intermediate to long duration of action

What non-benzodiazepine anxiolytic is used in the treatment of generalized anxiety disorder?

Buspirone, a serotonin-1A receptor partial agonist

What benefits does buspirone offer compared to benzodiazepine anxiolytics?

Minimal side effects and decreased potential for tolerance, dependence, and abuse

What benzodiazepine, marketed under the trade name Librium, is often used to treat severe alcohol withdrawal?	Chlordiazepoxide
Why is chlordiazepoxide preferred in the treatment of severe alcohol withdrawal?	Long duration of action and parenteral administration
What benefits does oxazepam offer compared to chlordiazepoxide in the treatment of severe alcohol withdrawal?	Renal elimination; and can be used in severe hepatic dysfunction
Why are diazepam and lorazepam preferred in the treatment of status epilepticus?	Rapid onset and parenteral administration
Why is the phenobarbital the preferred barbiturate in the maintenance treatment of seizure disorders?	Long duration of action
Why are oxazepam, temazepam, and triazolam the preferred benzodiazepines used in the acute treatment of insomnia?	Short duration of action
What non-benzodiazepine hypnotics are used in the acute treatment of insomnia?	Eszopiclone, zaleplon, and zolpidem
What benefits do eszopiclone, zaleplon, and zolpidem offer compared to benzodiazepine hypnotics?	Allow normal sleep patterns; and decreased potential for tolerance, dependence, and abuse
What benzodiazepine and barbiturate are used in the induction and maintenance of anesthesia?	Midazolam (shortest duration of action benzodiazepine) and thiopental (short duration of action barbiturate)

OPIOIDS

What peptides are the endogenous opioids of the CNS?	β-endorphin, dynorphin, and enkephalin
What CNS receptors are preferentially activated by β-endorphin, dynorphin, and enkephalin?	μ-, κ-, and δ-opioid receptors, respectively
What are the effects of opioids on the CNS?	Analgesia, euphoria, sedation, and respiratory depression

What are the clinical indications for administration of opioids?	Analgesia, anesthesia, pulmonary edema, cough suppression, and diarrhea
Why are opioids contraindicated in pulmonary dysfunction other than pulmonary edema?	Opioids depress respiratory drive.
Why are opioids contraindicated in states of increased intracranial pressure?	Opioids increase cerebrovascular dilation.
What are common side effects of opioids?	Respiratory depression, constipation, miosis, hypotension, and bradycardia
What are the effects of chronic opioid use?	Pharmacodynamic tolerance (except for constipation and miosis) and physical and psychological dependence
Which μ-opioid receptor agonists produce the strongest analgesic effect?	Fentanyl, levorphanol, meperidine, and morphine
What is the mechanism of action of morphine-induced hypotension?	Peripheral histamine release
Why is methadone preferred in the treatment of opioid addiction?	Enteral administration and long duration of action
Which μ-opioid receptor agonists produce a moderate analgesic effect?	Codeine, hydrocodone, and oxycodone
How does buprenorphine, a partial μ- opioid receptor agonist, produce strong analgesic effect?	Long duration of action due to high affinity for μ-opioid receptor
What agents are considered mixed opioid agonist-antagonists?	Butorphanol, nalbuphine, and pentazocine
What benefits do mixed opioid agonist-antagonists offer compared to full opioid agonists?	Minimal respiratory depression; and decreased potential for tolerance, dependence, and abuse
Why do mixed opioid agonist-antagonists produce less respiratory depression, tolerance, and dependence?	Strong agonist activity at κ-receptor and weak agonist activity at μ-receptor
What antitussive opioids are used in the treatment of cough?	Codeine and dextromethorphan
What opioids are used in the treatment of diarrhea?	Diphenoxylate and loperamide

What agents exhibit antagonist activity at μ-opioid receptors?	Naloxone, naltrexone, and nalmefene
What are the clinical indications for μ-opioid-receptor antagonists?	Acute treatment of opioid toxicity (naloxone, nalmefene) and maintenance of abstinence from alcohol (naltrexone)
What is the effect of opioid antagonist administration in opioid-tolerant individuals?	Provocation of opioid abstinence syndrome (withdrawal)

LOCAL ANESTHETICS

What is the desired effect of local anesthetics?	Prevention of transmission of local sensory stimuli to the CNS
What is the mechanism of action of the local anesthetics?	Inhibition of voltage-gated sodium ion channels
What is the site of action of local anesthetic?	Cytoplasm of neuronal axons
What chemical property influences diffusion of local anesthetic into neuronal axons?	Ionization status
Why are higher doses of local anesthetic required in acidic environments, eg, local infection and systemic acidosis?	Ionization of weakly basic local anesthetics impairs diffusion
Why do local anesthetics preferentially affect rapidly firing nerve fibers (use dependence)?	Preferential inhibition of open or recently inactivated ion channels
What physical characteristics of nerve fibers increase sensitivity to local anesthesia?	Smaller diameter and myelination
What are the two principal classes of local anesthetics?	Amides and esters
Which local anesthetics have a short duration of action?	Procaine and benzocaine (esters only)
Which local anesthetics have an intermediate duration of action?	Amides: lidocaine, mepivacaine, and prilocaine Ester: cocaine

Which local anesthetics have a long duration of action?

Amides: bupivacaine, etidocaine, and ropivacaine

Ester: tetracaine

How does the metabolism of local anesthetics influence their duration of action?

Esters rapidly metabolized by plasma cholinesterases; amides undergo hepatic metabolism.

Why does administration of epinephrine increase the duration of action of local anesthetics?

Vasoconstriction limits local blood flow, preventing systemic redistribution.

What are the CNS side effects of local anesthetics?

Light-headedness, nystagmus, restlessness, and seizure

What are the cardiovascular side effects of local anesthetics?

Bradycardia and hypotension (especially bupivacaine)

Tachycardia and hypertension (cocaine only)

What is the mechanism of action of allergic reaction to ester local anesthetics?

Para-aminobenzoic acid (PABA) formation

GENERAL ANESTHETICS

What is the pharmacokinetic significance of the solubility of inhalational general anesthetics?

Inversely proportional to duration of induction and recovery

How is solubility of inhalational general anesthetics quantified?

Blood/gas partition coefficient

What is the minimum alveolar concentration (MAC)?

Alveolar concentration of inhalational general anesthetic required to produce anesthesia in 50% of individuals

For what pharmacodynamic property is MAC a proxy?

Median effective dose (ED50)

What is the pharmacodynamic significance of the MAC of inhalational general anesthetics?

Inversely proportional to potency

How is the effect of anesthesia terminated?

Redistribution from the brain to the blood

Why is nitrous oxide unsuitable for single-agent anesthesia?	Low potency
What general anesthetic causes pulmonary irritation?	Desflurane
What general anesthetic is proconvulsant?	Enflurane
What general anesthetic causes hepatitis and arrhythmia?	Halothane
What general anesthetic is nephrotoxic?	Methoxyflurane
What potentially-fatal side effect can occur with coadministration of inhalational general anesthetics and skeletal muscle relaxants?	Malignant hyperthermia
Mutations in which calcium channel are often associated with malignant hyperthermia?	Ryanodine receptor
What agent is used in the treatment of malignant hyperthermia?	Dantrolene
What is the mechanism of action of dantrolene, a peripherally-acting spasmolytic?	Inhibition of ryanodine receptor-mediated calcium release from sarcoplasmic reticulum
What is the other potentially-fatal clinical indication for treatment with dantrolene?	Neuroleptic malignant syndrome
What pharmacokinetic properties of midazolam (benzodiazepine), thiopental, and methohexital (barbiturates) permit their use in induction and maintenance of general anesthesia?	Parenteral administration and short duration of action
What agents are used for rapid induction of anesthesia?	Propofol and etomidate
Describe the action of ketamine:	Dissociative amnestic and analgesic without true anesthetic properties
What is the "emergence reaction" associated with ketamine?	Excitation and disorientation on termination of anesthesia
Upon which receptor does ketamine act as an antagonist?	N-methyl-D-aspartate (NMDA) receptor

SKELETAL MUSCLE RELAXANTS

What is the mechanism of action of neuromuscular blockers?	Inhibition of motor end-plate nicotinic acetylcholine (ACh) receptors
What two classes of neuromuscular blockers inhibit motor end-plate nicotinic receptors?	Non-depolarizing competitive antagonists and depolarizing agonists
How do depolarizing neuromuscular blockers initially inhibit the action of endogenous ACh?	Decreased affinity for acetylcholinesterase (AChE) results in preferential metabolism of ACh.
What is the effect of decreased AChE metabolism of depolarizing blockers at the motor end-plate?	Persistent depolarization of the motor end-plate
How do muscles respond to this persistent motor end-plate depolarization?	With fasciculations, impairing coordinated contraction (phase I block)
What is the effect of continuous fasciculations on muscle activity?	Insensitivity to endogenous ACh (phase II block)
What effect do acetylcholinesterase (AChE) inhibitors (neostigmine, physostigmine) have on non-depolarizing neuromuscular blockers?	Potentiation of non-depolarizing blockade
What effect do AChE inhibitors (neostigmine, physostigmine) have on depolarizing neuromuscular blockers?	Potentiation of phase I depolarization blockade, reversal of phase II desensitization blockade
Why do mivacurium (non-depolarizing neuromuscular blocker) and succinylcholine (depolarizing neuromuscular blocker) have short durations of action?	Rapid metabolism by plasma cholinesterase
Why is atracurium a safer non-depolarizing neuromuscular blocker in hepatic and renal dysfunction?	Undergoes spontaneous elimination
What side effects result from muscle breakdown caused by treatment with succinylcholine?	Hyperkalemia and myalgia

What centrally-acting spasmolytics are indicated for the treatment of excessive muscle tone due to CNS dysfunction, eg, cerebral palsy and multiple sclerosis?

Baclofen (GABA$_B$ receptor agonist) and diazepam (benzodiazepine)

What centrally-acting spasmolytic is indicated for the treatment of excessive muscle tone due to acute muscle injury?

Cyclobenzaprine

What is the mechanism of action of botulinum toxin, a peripherally-acting spasmolytic?

Inhibition of ACh release from presynaptic vesicles

ANTIPSYCHOTICS

What hypothetical alteration in neurochemistry may be primarily responsible for the symptoms of psychotic disorders?

Functional mesolimbic/mesocortical dopamine excess (dopamine hypothesis of schizophrenia)

What is the mechanism of action of the typical antipsychotics?

Inhibition of D2 receptors of the mesolimbic/mesocortical pathways

What is the mechanism of typical antipsychotic-associated hyperprolactinemia?

Inhibition of D2 receptors of the tuberoinfundibular pathway

What are the early-onset, reversible extrapyramidal side effects associated with typical antipsychotics?

Dystonia, parkinsonism, and akathisia

What is the late-onset and irreversible extrapyramidal side effect associated with typical antipsychotics?

Tardive dyskinesia

How can treatment with benztropine help in distinguishing reversible and irreversible extrapyramidal side effects?

Reversible extrapyramidal side effects improve and tardive dyskinesia worsens with anticholinergics.

What is the treatment for typical antipsychotic-associated tardive dyskinesia?

Decrease or discontinue typical antipsychotic, switch to atypical.

Why do high-potency typical antipsychotics (haloperidol, fluphenazine) increase extrapyramidal side effects?

High affinity for D2 receptors inhibits dopamine activity in the nigrostriatal pathway at low doses.

Why do low-potency typical antipsychotics (chlorpromazine, thioridazine) increase nonspecific side effects?

Low affinity for D2 receptors requires higher therapeutic doses.

What nonspecific side effects associated with typical antipsychotics are attributable to anti-α-adrenergic effect?

Orthostatic hypotension and sexual dysfunction

What nonspecific side effects associated with typical antipsychotics are attributable to anticholinergic effect?

Constipation, dry mouth, urinary retention, and visual disturbances

What nonspecific side effects associated with typical antipsychotics are attributable to antihistamine effect?

Sedation and weight gain

What potentially-fatal side effect is associated with the use of typical antipsychotics?

Neuroleptic malignant syndrome

What are the symptoms of neuroleptic malignant syndrome?

Muscle rigidity, hyperthermia, and autonomic instability

What is the treatment of neuroleptic malignant syndrome?

Dantrolene, dopamine agonists, and supportive care

What is the mechanism of action of the atypical antipsychotics risperidone, olanzapine, quetiapine, ziprasidone, and aripiprazole?

5-HT2 receptor inhibition, weak D2 receptor inhibition

What is the mechanism of action of the atypical antipsychotic clozapine?

5-HT2 receptor inhibition, weak D4 receptor inhibition

What benefits do the atypical antipsychotics offer compared to the typical antipsychotics in the treatment of schizophrenia?

Improvement in both positive and negative symptoms and decreased extrapyramidal side effects

What serious hematologic side effect associated with clozapine?

Agranulocytosis

What electrocardiogram changes are associated with ziprasidone?

Prolonged QT interval and torsade de pointes

Which atypical antipsychotic is most likely to be associated with extrapyramidal side effects?

Risperidone

ANTIDEPRESSANTS

To what alteration in neurochemistry are symptoms of affective disorders typically attributed?	Functional norepinephrine and serotonin deficiency (biogenic amine theory of depression)
What antidepressant drug class includes amitriptyline, imipramine, nortriptyline, and desipramine?	Tricyclic antidepressants
What is the mechanism of action of the tricyclic antidepressants?	Nonselective inhibition of presynaptic norepinephrine and serotonin reuptake
What drug class has a side effect profile similar to that of the tricyclic antidepressants?	Low-potency typical antipsychotics
What side effects associated with tricyclic antidepressants are attributable to anti-α-adrenergic, anticholinergic, and antihistamine effects?	Orthostatic hypotension, sexual dysfunction, constipation, dry mouth, urinary retention, visual disturbances, sedation, and weight gain
What are the symptoms of tricyclic antidepressant toxicity?	Coma, convulsion, cardiotoxicity (three Cs), mydriasis, and hyperthermia
How is tricyclic antidepressant toxicity best treated?	Cyproheptadine or benzodiazepines for seizure, anti-arrhythmics, and supportive care
What antidepressant drug class includes amoxapine, bupropion, maprotiline, trazodone, mirtazapine, nefazodone, and venlafaxine?	Heterocyclic antidepressants
Which heterocyclic antidepressant is most likely to be associated with priapism and sedation?	Trazodone
Which heterocyclic antidepressants are most likely to be associated with seizure and cardiotoxicity?	Amoxipine and maprotiline
Which heterocyclic antidepressant is most likely to be associated with extrapyramidal side effects?	Amoxipine
Which heterocyclic antidepressants are associated with cytochrome P450 enzyme inhibition?	Nefazodone and venlafaxine

Which heterocyclic antidepressant is used in the treatment of nicotine addiction?	Bupropion
What antidepressant drug class includes citalopram, fluoxetine, fluvoxamine, paroxetine, and sertraline?	Selective serotonin reuptake inhibitors (SSRIs)
What is the mechanism of action of the SSRIs?	Selective inhibition of presynaptic serotonin reuptake
What are the common side effects of SSRIs?	Anxiety, insomnia, nausea, and sexual dysfunction
What are the symptoms of SSRI toxicity?	Agitation, confusion, coma, muscle rigidity, hyperthermia, seizure, and autonomic instability
How is SSRI toxicity best treated?	Cyproheptadine or benzodiazepine for seizure, and supportive care
What antidepressant drug class includes phenelzine, tranylcypromine, and isocarboxazid?	Monoamine oxidase (MAO) inhibitors
What is the mechanism of action of the MAO inhibitors?	Nonselective inhibition of metabolism of serotonin, norepinephrine, and dopamine by MAO-A and MOA-B
What are the common side effects of MAO inhibitors?	Orthostatic hypotension, insomnia, and weight gain
What drugs can provoke a hypertensive crisis when coadministered with MAO inhibitors?	Indirect-acting sympathomimetics (cocaine, amphetamine) and tyramine (red wine, aged cheese)
What are the symptoms associated with serotonin syndrome?	Muscle rigidity, hyperthermia, autonomic instability, and seizure
Coadministration of which drugs is associated with serotonin syndrome?	SSRIs, tricyclic antidepressants, MAO inhibitors, meperidine, and/or dextromethorphan
What drugs are indicated in the first-line treatment of bipolar disorders?	Lithium, valproic acid, and olanzapine
What is the mechanism of action of lithium in the treatment of bipolar disorders?	Inhibition of neuronal phosphoinositide recycling
Why are atypical antipsychotics and/or benzodiazepines indicated in the initial treatment of bipolar disorders?	Lithium has slow onset of action.

What hematologic side effect is associated with lithium?	Leukocytosis
What reversible renal side effect is associated with lithium?	Nephrogenic diabetes insipidus
Why does the plasma concentration of lithium have to be monitored regularly?	Lithium has a narrow therapeutic index.
What is the therapeutic index?	Ratio of the median toxic (TD50) or lethal (LD50) dose to the median effective dose (ED50)

PHARMACOLOGIC TREATMENT OF PARKINSON DISEASE

What alteration of neurochemistry is responsible for the symptoms of parkinsonism and Parkinson disease?	Dopamine deficiency and/or ACh excess in the striatum
What is the mechanism of action of L-dopa?	Synthetic precursor converted to dopamine by DOPA decarboxylase.
How does coadministration of carbidopa increase the potency of L-dopa?	Inhibition of peripheral conversion of L-dopa to dopamine
What chemical property of carbidopa is responsible for preferential inhibition of peripheral L-dopa metabolism?	Poor lipid solubility prevents diffusion across blood-brain barrier.
What other peripheral enzyme inhibitors enhance the potency of L-dopa?	Entacapone and tolcapone
What is the mechanism of action of entacapone?	Inhibition of peripheral conversion of L-dopa to 3-O-methyldopa by catecholamine-O-methyltransferase (COMT)
What is the mechanism of action of pramipexole, a first-line treatment in the initial management of Parkinson disease?	Direct activation of D2 receptor in the striatum
To what drug class do the antiparkinson medications bromocriptine and pergolide belong?	Ergot alkaloids
What are the symptoms of ergotism toxicity (St. Anthony's fire)?	Disorientation, hallucination, convulsion, muscle cramps, and dry gangrene of extremities

What drug of abuse is an ergot alkaloid?

Lysergic acid diethylamide (LSD)

Why is selegiline, a selective MAO-B inhibitor, an effective treatment for parkinsonism?

MAO-B is CNS-specific and preferentially metabolizes dopamine

What is the mechanism of action of antiparkinsonian agents benztropine and trihexyphenidyl?

Inhibition of the striatum muscarinic anticholinergic receptors

PHARMACOLOGIC TREATMENT OF ALZHEIMER DISEASE

What alteration in neurochemistry is the basis for current therapeutics in Alzheimer disease?

Functional cortical and hippocampal ACh deficiency

What class of drug is indicated in the treatment of mild to moderate Alzheimer disease?

AChE inhibitors, eg, rivastigmine, donepezil, galantamine, and tacrine

What is the mechanism of action of the AChE inhibitors in the treatment of Alzheimer disease?

Increased concentration of synaptic terminal ACh

What other enzyme is inhibited by rivastigmine and tacrine?

Butyrylcholinesterase

What drug class is indicated in the treatment of moderate to severe Alzheimer disease?

NMDA antagonists (memantine)

What is the mechanism of action of the NMDA antagonists in the treatment of Alzheimer disease?

Inhibition of glutaminergic NMDA calcium conductance

DRUGS OF ABUSE

What is tolerance?

Habituation to the physiologic effects of a drug

What are the pharmacodynamic effects of tolerance?

It decreases efficacy and larger doses are required to achieve the same effect.

What is dependence?

A physiologic and/or psychologic state characterized by compulsive substance use

What are the effects of alcohol intoxication?	Increased sociability and impairment of motor, cognitive, and memory function
What is the mechanism of action of alcohol intoxication?	Incompletely understood, GABAergic and generalized CNS depression
How is alcohol metabolized?	Via a two-step process with zero-order kinetics and a toxic intermediate
What is the first step in metabolism of alcohol?	Conversion of alcohol to acetaldehyde by cytoplasmic alcohol dehydrogenase
What is the second step in metabolism of alcohol?	Conversion of acetaldehyde to acetate by mitochondrial aldehyde dehydrogenase
What are the effects of acetaldehyde toxicity?	Nausea, vomiting, hyperventilation, tachycardia, chest pain, and dyspnea
What agent used in the treatment of alcohol dependence inhibits aldehyde dehydrogenase causing acetaldehyde accumulation?	Disulfiram
What is the hypothesized mechanism of action of acamprosate in the treatment of alcohol dependence?	Relapse prevention via decreased glutamate receptor sensitivity
What is the mechanism of action of benzodiazepine in the treatment of alcohol dependence?	Withdrawal seizure treatment and prophylaxis via $GABA_A$ receptor activation
What is the mechanism of action of naltrexone in the treatment of alcohol dependence?	Reduces cravings via opioid receptor inhibition
What are the symptoms of acute alcohol withdrawal?	Agitation, tremor, insomnia, nausea, vomiting, diarrhea, arrhythmia, delirium tremens, and potentially-fatal seizure
What is the treatment for acute alcohol withdrawal?	Thiamine, benzodiazepine taper, clonidine, and propranolol for hyperadrenergic state
What other CNS depressants are frequently abused?	Benzodiazepines and barbiturates
What are the symptoms of CNS depressant withdrawal?	Agitation, delirium, insomnia, and potentially-fatal seizure

What drugs are indicated in the treatment of CNS depressant withdrawal?	Long-acting benzodiazepine to suppress acute symptoms, tapering dose
What drugs are indicated in the treatment of CNS depressant toxicity?	Flumazenil for benzodiazepine toxicity
What is the mechanism of action of CNS stimulants?	Increased synaptic terminal concentration of dopamine, norepinephrine, and serotonin
What are the symptoms of CNS stimulant intoxication?	Euphoria, anxiety, insomnia, anorexia, tachycardia, hypertension, and mydriasis
What are the symptoms of CNS stimulant withdrawal?	Depression, fatigue, increased sleep, and increased appetite
What are the symptoms of CNS stimulant toxicity?	Arrhythmia, MI, cardiovascular, hallucination, paranoia, hyperthermia, seizure, and death
What drugs are indicated in the treatment of CNS stimulant toxicity?	Benzodiazepine and antipsychotic agents
What are the symptoms of opioid intoxication?	Euphoria, analgesia, cough suppression, miosis, and constipation
What are the symptoms of opioid withdrawal?	Mydriasis, diarrhea, rhinorrhea, lacrimation, diaphoresis, and yawning
What drugs are indicated in the treatment of opioid withdrawal?	Methadone, LAAM, buprenorphine, and clonidine
What are the symptoms of opioid toxicity?	Nausea, vomiting, sedation, respiratory depression, bradycardia, hypotension, coma, and death
What drugs are indicated in the treatment of opioid toxicity?	Naloxone and naltrexone
What is the mechanism of action of cannabis (marijuana, hashish) intoxication?	Cannabinoid (CB1 and CB2) receptor activation
What are the symptoms of cannabis intoxication?	Euphoria, disinhibition, perceptual changes, conjunctival injection, dry mouth, and increased appetite

What is the mechanism of action of hallucinogens (LSD, mescaline, psilocybin) intoxication?	Serotonin receptor activation
What are the symptoms of hallucinogen intoxication?	Perceptual changes and synesthesia
What are the symptoms of hallucinogen withdrawal?	No physiologic dependence
What is the mechanism of action of phencyclidine (PCP; "angel dust")?	NMDA receptor antagonist
What are the symptoms of PCP intoxication?	Agitation, nystagmus, rigidity, decreased response to pain, hyperacusis, paranoia, and violent behavior
What is the mechanism of action of 3,4-methylenedioxymethamphetamine (MDMA; "ecstasy") intoxication?	Increased synaptic terminal concentration of serotonin
What are the symptoms of MDMA intoxication?	Euphoria, disinhibition, and perceptual changes
What are the symptoms of inhalant (glue, solvents) toxicity?	Motor and cognitive impairment and multiple organ dysfunction

CLINICAL VIGNETTES

Make the diagnosis for the following patients:

A 24-year-old man with recent onset of schizophrenia is brought to the ER and presents with tachycardia, tachypnea, diaphoresis, rigid muscles, incontinence, and a fever of 42°C. Despite development of newer atypical antipsychotics, the patient was started on an older typical antipsychotic, haloperidol, 2 weeks ago. Labs reveal leukocytosis, metabolic acidosis, as well as elevated creatinine phosphokinase (CPK) and urinary myoglobin.

Neuroleptic malignant syndrome

A 32-year-old man was under inhaled general anesthetic for a minor surgical procedure when the operating room staff noticed increasing muscle rigidity and tachycardia. They also found that the patient's temperature had increased to 41°C and his serum CO_2 was 35 mmol/L. The anesthesia team administered dantrolene. Lab tests later revealed elevated CPK, potassium, and urinary myoglobin.

Malignant hyperthermia

A 43-year-old man well-known to the ER staff as a chronic alcohol abuser is brought in by ambulance after a witnessed seizure. Witnesses also reported the man was unsteady, vomiting, and appeared agitated, confused, and described visual hallucinations. On physical examination, the patient remains confused and agitated, and is ataxic, tremulous, tachycardic, diaphoretic, and mydriatic; and has a blood pressure of 145/100 mm Hg. Blood tests reveal increased AST, ALT, and GGT. Diazepam is administered following a subsequent seizure, after which time the patient is maintained on chlordiazepoxide.

Delirium tremens (Alcohol withdrawal)

Suggested Readings

Afifi AH, Bergman RA. *Functional Neuroanatomy.* 2nd ed. New York, NY: McGraw Hill; 2005.

Berne RM, Levy MN, Koeppen BM, et al. *Physiology.* 5th ed. St Louis, MO: Mosby; 2003.

Cotran RS, Kumar V, Collins T, et al. *Robbins Pathologic Basis of Disease.* 6th ed. Philadelphia, PA: W.B. Saunders; 1999.

Kandel ER, Schwartz JH, Jessell TM. *Principles of Neural Science.* 4th ed. New York, NY: McGraw-Hill; 2000.

Katzung BG. *Basic and Clinical Pharmacology.* 9th ed. New York, NY: McGraw-Hill; 2003.

Martin JH. *Neuroanatomy Text and Atlas.* 3rd ed. New York, NY: McGraw-Hill; 2003.

Ropper AH, Brown RH. *Adams and Victor's Principles of Neurology.* 8th ed. New York, NY: McGraw-Hill; 2005.

Index

Page numbers followed by *f* or *t* indicate figures or tables, respectively.

vitamin A, 204–205, 207
vitamin B$_1$, 127–128, 203
vitamin B$_6$, 159, 204
vitamin B$_{12}$, 18, 204
vitamin E, 204
von Hippel-Lindau syndrome, 151
von Recklinghausen disease. *See*
  neurofibromatosis type 1

W
Wallenberg syndrome, 35, 37*t*, 38*f*, 47, 138
Wallerian degeneration, 209
Weber syndrome, 36, 37*t*, 38*f*, 47, 138
Weber test, 87, 87*t*
Wegener granulomatosis, 212
Werdnig-Hoffman disease, 96, 198

Wernicke encephalopathy, 127–128, 203
Wernicke-Korsakoff syndrome, 192, 203
Wernicke aphasia, 58–59, 60*t*, 137
West syndrome, 179
Wilson disease, 104–105, 114
withdrawal, 228–231
working memory, 53, 185

X
xanthochromia, 139

Z
zaleplon, 216
ziprasidone, 223
zolpidem, 216
zonisamide, 181